Progress in Orthopaedic Surgery Vol. 1

Leg Length Discrepancy

The Injured Knee

Edited by David S. Hungerford

Contributors
W. Bandi, Interlaken · J. Eichler, Wiesbaden · G. Figner, Basel · P. Heidensohn, Erlangen · E. Hogue, Jackson · D. Hohmann, Erlangen · J. L. Hughes, Jackson · Ch. Kieser, Zurich · E. Meyer, Hanover · E. Morscher, Basel · W. Müller, Basel · D. Petersen, Hanover · A. Rüttimann, Zurich · H. Wagner, Nuremberg/Altdorf · M. Weigert, Erlangen

With 100 Figures

Springer-Verlag
Berlin Heidelberg New York 1977

Editor: David S. Hungerford, The Johns Hopkins University, School of Medicine, The Good Samaritan Hospital, 5601 Loch Raven Boulevard, Baltimore, Maryland 21239, USA.

ISBN-13: 978-3-642-66551-6 e-ISBN-13: 978-3-642-66549-3
DOI: 10.1007/978-3-642-66549-3

Library of Congress Cataloging in Publication Data. Leg length discrepancy. (Progress in orthopaedic surgery; v. 1) Consists chiefly of articles from Der Orthopäde, v. 1, 1972, and v. 3, 1974. Bibliography: p. Includes index. 1. Leg length inequality-Addresses, essays, lectures. 2. Knee-Wounds and injuries-Addresses, essays, lectures. I. Hungerford, David S. II. Bandi, W. III. Series. [DNLM: 1. Leg length inequality. 2. Knee injuries. Wl PR677B v. 1/WE850 L496] RD779.3.L43 617'.398 76-57743

Softcover reprint of the hardcover 1st edition 1977

Foreword by H. Wagner

Research worldwide in the field of orthopaedic surgery has resulted in such an abundance of scientific and technical knowledge that textbooks no longer can keep abreast of new developments while journals, on the other hand, fail to provide a comprehensive broad view.

To satisfy the orthopaedic surgeon's need for information, the German-language journal *Der Orthopäde* was founded in 1972. Since then, the journal has published the latest results of scientific research applicable to practice, and provided review papers which have also been of interest to those in allied specialities. This form of disseminating scientific knowledge has met with acceptance and found a wide circle of readers stretching beyond the boundaries of Europe. Many other orthopaedic surgeons have expressed an interest in the information contained in this publication but have found the language barrier insurmountable. A new series *Progress in Orthopaedic Surgery* has been created in order to make this information available. It will present both the work of European authors in English and also original papers from American orthopaedic surgeons.

Each volume will provide a broad overview of the current state of knowledge in one or two themes of orthopaedic surgery. The choice of themes will be decided by the editors with major emphasis on diagnosis, prevention, and treatment of orthopaedic disorders. The editors will call upon authorities in the field to supply these current reports.

It is the editors' wish that this new series will build bridges across language barriers and enrich the exchange of information in orthopaedic surgery.

Nuremberg/Altdorf December 1976

Foreword by David S. Hungerford

Two timely topics have been selected by the editors for the initial volume of the new series *Progress in Orthopaedic Surgery*. The series begins with primarily European contributions on a subject which is more prevalent in Europe than in many of the English speaking countries. It is therefore not surprising that significant advances have been achieved in the evaluation and treatment of significant leg length discrepancy based on the need to solve the associated complex technical problems. This section on leg length discrepancy comprehensively covers the problem from diagnosis, methods of quantifying discrepancy, and pathomechanics to non-surgical and surgical treatment of the discrepancy. Recognized experts in the field have concisely presented their experience. Together these articles comprise a section which represents the "state of the art" for evaluation and treatment of leg length discrepancy.

The second topic deals with the injured knee. Dr. Müller presents a comprehensive overview of the soccer player's knee. With the growing interest and involvement of this sport in the United States involving all age groups, this article will be particularly appreciated. Professors Bandi and Wagner deal with the question of cartilage injury in the knee. Certainly such lesions occur more frequently than they are diagnosed. Professor Bandi brings his long-standing interest and experience in patella pathology to bear on the question of a traumatic etiology of chondromalacia patellae. Professor Wagner elucidates a variety of kinds of cartilage injury, both direct and indirect, with practical suggestions for diagnosis and treatment.

The first volume of *Progress in Orthopaedic Surgery* has been edited to introduce English-speaking orthopaedists to the works and thinking of their German-speaking colleagues. Outstanding work on timely topics has been selected with the hope that this series will provide a common ground for communication between these two important language groups.

Baltimore December 1976

Contents

Leg Length Discrepancy

Basic Rehabilitation Principles of Persons with Leg Length Discrepancy: An Overview

J. L. Hughes* and R. E. Hogue**

A sucessful rehabilitation program is built upon a thorough evaluation of the patient's physical and emotional problems. A person with leg length discrepancy may have functional, cosmetic, or pain problems. Proper identification of these problems is imperative if the treatment is to bear desired results. It is necessary for the physician and therapists to work with the patient in a team approach from the very beginning. The team approach enables the proper priorities to be placed on the problem areas; to try to correct all problem areas at once would be futile. For some patients cosmesis is the overriding factor in their desire to have corrective measures performed. In others, function may be the most inportant factor. Some defects may be minor to the evaluators but major to the patient, or vice versa.

Once the initial team evaluation is accomplished, a therapy program should be planned and implemented whether it be surgical, conservative, or both. Implementation of the treatment program should not mean the end of the evaluation. Evaluation is an ongoing process until there is mutual satisfaction by the evaluators and the patients. Ongoing evaluation also enables the examiners to determine the success of the treatment program and make necessary modifications if the need should arise.

Evaluation of the patient with leg length discrepancy should be centered in four major areas. In all of these areas of investigation the findings should be properly recorded so that an adequate data base may be obtained for making future decisions and for comparing future analysis. Initially, one should look at the affected limb in order to ascertain the etiology of the leg length discrepancy. This includes a thorough evaluation of the neuromuscular components of the extremity, as well as the joints that are incorporated in the extremity. Attention

* Chairman, Division of Orthopaedic Surgery, University of Mississippi Medical School, Jackson, Mississippi, USA
** Chairman, Department of Physical Therapy, School of Related Health Professions, University of Mississippi School of Medicine, and Chairman, Physical Therapy & Kinesiology, Mississippi Methodist Rehabilitation Center

should be paid to the soft tissues and their probable contracted state. One should also look at the sound leg in as thorough a manner as the affected side. The pelvis, and thoracic and lumbar spine must be evaluated to determine their functional and anatomical state. Lastly, a thorough knowledge of the patient's attitude and desires should be obtained, for if there are major defects in these areas even the most skilled rehabilitation program will fail. Once these basic premises are understood, the thorough evaluation can proceed.

Many of the factors mentioned in this article will be reviewed in greater detail by the other participants in this volume. However, this overview will provide the framework within which that detail can be placed.

A complete evaluation program of the patient with a leg length discrepancy should include the following measurements.

Leg Length

Measurement of the leg length should be done in supine, standing, and sitting positions. These are the functional positions which are most frequently used during the day. One method of measuring the leg length is from the anterior superior iliac spine to the medial malleolus, or from the anterior superior iliac spine to the tip of the lateral malleolus. This is done with the patient in a supine position. Each segment of the lower extremity should also be measured. In the standing position, one should have several thicknesses of boards available to determine the functional discrepancy of the shortened leg. These boards should be inserted between the sole of the foot and the floor until the pelvis becomes level. This is accomplished by the observer viewing the iliac crest posteriorly. A gross measurement of pelvic obliquity can be obtained by measuring from the patient's umbilicus to the anterior superior iliac spine. Even though the clinical measurements are important, they cannot take the place of an adequately controlled radiologic study of the pelvis and the lower extremities to determine the absolute leg length discrepancy.

Circumference

Measurements should be accomplished about the thigh approximately 8 to 10 inches above the tibial tubercle and around the calf approximately 6 to 8 inches below the tibial tubercle. These measurements determine differences in the contralateral muscle mass and, in addition, can be used as a guide to determine the results of the strengthening exercises.

Strength

The patient's strength should be tested manually at all joints of the lower extremities and, in addition, the anterior and posterior spinal and abdominal muscles should be tested. A percentage, numerical, or letter system may be used to assign grades. Documenting the muscle strength will assist the surgeon in making decisions about the need for surgery. The manual muscle test will also assist in determining whether the patient needs assistive devices and will aid in the effectiveness of the treatment program, especially if muscle tests are done in a serial fashion.

Range of Motion

Range of motion should be checked with a goniometer and done against gravity. If there is a limitation of joint motion, the examiner must determine if this is due to weakness of the agonist muscle, tightness or contracture of the antagonist muscle, bony defects, adhesions, or a degenerative joint disease process.

Posture Examination

The patient should be completely unclothed, and a marking pencil should be used to mark the spinous processes, borders and angles of the scapulae, anterior superior iliac spine, iliac crest, posterior superior iliac spine, patellae, greater trochanters, and the navicular bone of the foot. This posture examination will determine if the patient has scoliosis, pelvic tilt, genu varus or valgus, pronation or supination of the foot, pes planus or pes cavus. As part of this examination, the patient's coordination and balance should be checked. Depending on the patient's physical abnormalities, coordination may be checked by doing bilateral symmetrical exercises such as running in place, riding a bicycle, et cetera. The patient's balance should be able to take resistance while sitting with the back unsupported and to stand on the sound leg without support. Obesity is detrimental to any successful rehabilitation effort and should be corrected.

The evaluation must include a complete gait analysis. After the initial examination, each joint should be looked at separately. A person with a short limb may reveal a gait similar to that of a gluteus medius weakness. The opposite pelvis may drop while the patient is in the stance phase on the affected side, or the patient may compensate by leaning sharply to the affected side in the frontal plane. Other gait deviations may be manifested because of tightness, weakness, contractures, pain, hysterical causes, peripheral nerve injuries, or because of affectation of the upper motor neurons. In addition to observing the phases and subdivisions of gait, the patient's step length, stride length, step width, cadence and timing should be checked. Any patient with a significant leg length discrepancy will show abnormalities in the width, timing, and length measurements.

Pain and Sensation

Evaluation of pain depends primarily on the patient's description, although a general idea can be obtained by palpating the affected area or through range of motion testing. Sensation should always be tested. In some patients compression of a peripheral nerve or nerve root may occur.

Functional Activities

Specific muscle and joint testings are important but the most significant thing to the patient is the ability to function. If the patient cannot perform activities of daily living adequately within the least amount of time, training is necessary.

Special Testing Procedures

Surface or intramuscular electromyography may be used to determine the specific function of muscles during gait, muscle testing, or with other functional activities. In cases of suspected myopathy or neuropathy, electromyography and nerve conduction studies may be necessary. Thermograms are used to determine the temperature differential over a joint or any suspected area of inflammation. The electrogoniometers are utilized over the hip, knee, and ankle during gait to allow accurate measurements for determining the effectiveness of any surgical procedures or conservative regimens in improving functional motion. Foot switches may also be used in analyzing gait, serving to determine a pattern of foot contact with the floor. Telemetry can transport the foot switch signals to a computer or paper recorder.

After the various examinations are accomplished and recorded, a customized program of rehabilitation can be outlined for each patient. It should be emphasized that each program should be individualized. Each patient has his individual anatomical, emotional, and functional needs. At this point in the evaluation, a plan can be formulated by the surgeon and the team regarding conservative versus surgical treatment which would include an adequate rehabilitation program.

If complete documentation reveals a limb length discrepancy of less than 2.5 cm, coupled with all other indicators pointing toward a conservative approach, the following guidelines may be utilized.

A properly fitted shoe, with the appropriate lifts placed either on the inner or outer sole, can be manufactured to create an extremity that is functionally equal in length to the opposite side. This must be coupled with a program of postural exercises for the thoracic and lumbar spine. In addition, exercises directed toward correcting any pelvic obliquity should be given the patient. Active resistive exercises to strengthen the quadriceps and hamstrings, as well as the musculature about both hips, should be undertaken on a daily basis. The patient should not be discharged from care until his gait is normalized and maintained over a period of 3 to 6 months. In many cases, long-standing, poor gait habits necessitate a long-term program for the necessary correction.

If the leg length discrepancy is greater than 2.5 cm, consideration should be given to surgical correction. Surgical correction falls into two major categories, i.e. shortening of the sound extremity, or lengthening of the shortened limb. There are advantages and disadvantages to both but, with the newer and stronger lengthening devices (Wagner apparatus), the lengthening procedures are becoming more and more common. If the patient is given a montage showing his present status, the long limb shortened, or the shorter limb lengthened, he will in most cases choose to lengthen the shorter limb. This may, in the case of a severe shortening, necessitate several lengthening procedures. With a great deal of shortening, there are usually superimposed problems such as contractures of the gastrosoleus group, knee flexors and adductors and, quite possibly, the hip flexors, abductors and adductors. Prior to any surgical program an educational process is carried out so that the patient fully understands the surgical procedure. With the newer appliances, such as the Wagner apparatus for lengthening and the AO plates utilized for shortening, the patient has the responsibility for absolute pre- and postsurgical cooperation. Any misunderstanding involving the patient's use of the operated extremity can bring disastrous results to the total rehabilitation program. All of the surgical techniques presently employed allow active motion of the joints, proximal and distal to the operative site, which enables the patient to continue his active rehabilitation program postoperatively.

Prior to surgery, active resistive exercises should be accomplished in all muscle groups with an emphasis on the hip abductors and extensors. The quadriceps and hamstrings should also be strengthened to their maximum capabilities. Postoperatively, active motion is allowed if the surgeon designates that adequate stabilization of the osteotomy site has been accomplished by the implant or external fixative device. Active exercise of all joints is to be encouraged, but no resistive exercise or passive manipulation can be tolerated. The patient is allowed only toe touch weight bearing. When satisfactory bone healing has been determined, resistive exercises to further strengthen the muscles can be undertaken. In many cases after surgery, it is necessary to manually stretch the muscles that have been shortened and to teach the proper exercises for strengthening the antagonistic muscles. Continued stretching exercises should be carried out for the adjacent joints that reveal soft tissue restrictions.

Attention should be given to active exercises, in the immediate postoperative and late phase, for strengthening the lumbar spine and pelvis. Exercises necessary for strengthening the upper extremities should also be carried out.

Any patient with a leg length discrepancy will benefit from gait training. Proper instruction both pre- and postoperatively will assist the patient in breaking old habits and forming new ones. Instruction before a mirror will assist the patient in the proper step and stride length, width, cadence and timing. A smooth gait will be advantageous from an energy viewpoint, as well as markedly improve his cosmesis.

The team must be realistic in determining goals for gait training. Some patients have to be satisfied with less than a desirable gait pattern. The gait training process is greatly enhanced if there has been a proper program of exercises for those muscles which have been weak, and stretching exercises for muscles which have been shortened. Weak muscles, made to work frequently and too long in walking and other varied activities, will tend to become weaker. It may be necessary, at least on a short-term basis, to utilize assistive devices until these muscles develop to their maximum strength. A cane may be utilized for balance.

Summary

A successful rehabilitation program is built upon a thorough evaluation of the patient's physical and emotional problems. The tests and measurements to be performed in evaluating a patient with leg length discrepancy have been enumerated and briefly described. Examples of treatment programs have been given, and should be based on the needs of the patient after completion of the initial and subsequent evaluations. The key to the success of a treatment program, either pre- or postsurgically, is based upon a sound therapeutic exercise program including strengthening, stretching, and gait training. Other treatment procedures include assistive devices such as the proper shoes, shoe lifts, canes and crutches.

References

Daniels, L., Worthingham, C.: Muscle Testing, Philadelphia, PA: W. B. Saunders, 1972
Hogue, R. E.: Upper-extremity muscular activity at different cadences and inclines during normal gait. J. Amer. Phys. Ther. Ass. **49,** 963–972 (1969)
Müller, M. F., Allgöwer, M., Willenegger, H.: Manual of Internal Fixation **VII** (1970)
Saunders, J. B., Inman, V. T. Eberhart, H. D.: The major determinants in normal and pathological gait. Journal of Bone & Joint Surgery **35 A** 543–558 (1953)
Steindler, A.: Kinesiology of the Human Body, Springfield, ILL: Charles C Thomas, 1955
Wagner, H.: Personal communication
Wells, K. F.: Kinesiology. Philadelphia, PA: W. B. Saunders, 1976

Etiology and Pathophysiology of Leg Length Discrepancies

E. Morscher*

Measuring and correcting leg length discrepancies are part of the everyday activities of the orthopaedist, yet these activities are hardly mentioned in orthopaedic textbooks. One gets the impression that nothing is easier than to measure these discrepancies, to lengthen the shorter leg by prescribing a shoe lift or to shorten a longer one with an osteotomy. Yet the problem of unequal leg length is undoubtedly more complex. Any artifical change in leg length interferes with the extremely delicate compensating mechanisms of statics and dynamics of the locomotor system, of which there has been all too little investigation. This is particularly true at the level of the intervertebral disc. Therefore every correction of leg length discrepancy must be preceded by an accurate analysis of its etiology and its clinical consequences.

1. Etiology of Leg Length Discrepancies

One has to distinguish between true discrepancies caused by shortening or lengthening of a single or several bones, and functional changes usually caused by joint contractures or other deformities. The numerous causes of true leg length discrepancies are summarized in Table 1.

Until recently, poliomyelitis was the most common cause of leg length discrepancies. This resulted in marked differences in length, generally requiring surgical correction. In 1957 Ratliff reported only six poliomyelitis patients out of 225 without shortening of their lower extremities. Today most leg length differences of a more severe nature are caused by congenital abnormalities such as femoral hypoplasia or congenital hemihypertrophy. Epiphyseal plate injuries with subsequent growth disturbance may also lead to significant limb shortening.

Fractures in children are a particular problem. It is well known that hyperemia due to fracture healing results in stimulation of the growth activity of the corresponding epiphyseal plate. Blount has stated repeatedly that childrens' fractures

* Orthopädische Universitätsklinik Basel, Basel, Switzerland

Table 1. Causes of leg length discrepancies during the age of bone growth (from Taillard and Morscher)

	By growth retardation	By growth stimulation
I. Congenital	Congenital hemiatrophy with skeletal anomalies (fibular aplasia, femoral aplasia, coxa vara etc.), dyschondroplasia (Ollier's disease), dysplasia epiphysealis punctata, multiple exostoses, CDH; clubfoot	Partial giantism with vascular abnormalities (Klippel-Trenaunay, Parkes-Weber) Hemarthrosis due to hemophila
II. Infection	Epiphyseal plate destruction due to osteomyelitis (femur, tibia) tuberculosis (hip, knee joint, foot), septic arthritis	Diaphyseal osteomyelitis of femur or tibia, Brodie's abscess Metaphyseal tuberculosis of femur or tibia (tumor albus) Septic arthritis Syphilis of femur or tibia Elephantiasis as a result of soft tissue infections Thrombosis of femoral or iliac veins
III. Paralysis	Poliomyelitis, other paralysis (spastic)	
IV. Tumors	Osteochondroma (solitary exostosis) Giant cell tumors Osteitis fibrosa cystica generalisata Neurofibromatosis (Recklinghausen)	Hemangioma, lymphangioma Giant cell tumors Osteitis fibrosa cystica generalisato Neurofibromatosis Recklinghausen Fibrous dysplasia (Jaffe-Lichtenstein)
V. Trauma	Damage of the epiphyseal plate (dislocation, operation etc.) Diaphyseal fractures with marked overriding of fragments Severe burns	Dia- and metaphyseal fractures of femur or tibia (Osteosynthesis!) Diaphyseal operations (stripping of periosteum, bone graft removal osteotomy etc.)
VI. Mechanical	Immobilization of long duration by weight-relieving braces	Traumatic arteriovenous aneurysms
VII. Others	Legg-Calvé-Perthes' disease Slipped upper femoral epiphysis Damage to femoral or tibial epiphyseal plates due to radiation therapy	

should never be reduced in an ideal position but should be allowed to heal with some overriding of the fragments. In 1967 Staheli noted that the strongest growth stimulation occurs in femoral fractures of children between the age of 2 and 12 and recommended for this age group alignment of the fragments with 0.5 to 1.5 cm overriding.

Stimulation of activity of the epiphyseal plate corresponds to the amount and duration of the hyperemia. This is borne out by the observation of a considerable increase in bone length after internal fixation of fractures in children.

It is dangerous however to rely on epiphyseal plate stimulation as a factor of bone length in older children. Our observations have shown that at puberty – at a time shortly before the epiphyseal plate closes – the ossification process of the epiphyseal plate is enhanced, not the longitudinal bone growth. This can result in an early closure of the growth plate with corresponding shortening of the involved bone. There also remains an unanswered question. Is it possible that the factor(s) causing epiphyseal stimulation, whatever their nature, also unleash factors leading to epiphyseal closure? This would result in the once stimulated epiphysis closing earlier than would be expected.

Much more common than leg length discrepancies of many centimeters are lesser ones up to 2 cm. Their causes are, in most instances, unknown, rendering them truly idiopathic. Their true frequency remains in doubt since different figures have been recorded. In 1893 Hasse and Dehner reported the presence of leg length differences in 68% of 5141 soldiers. Rush and Steiner (1946) found discrepancies of a few millimeters to 2 cm in 71 of 100 healthy U.S. soldiers. Hult (1954) noted in 30% of Swedish laborers differences from 1.0 to 2.5 cm. The same author found, in a mixed population of 1137 individuals, discrepancies of 2.0 to 2.5 cm in 4.3%, between 3.0 and 4.5 cm in 0.7%. In 1959 Sollman examined 1016 patients and noted a pelvic tilt in 15% with leg length discrepancies above 10 mm.

In 1957 Edinger and Biedermann examined 325 individuals radiologically. They found a difference of less than 5 mm in 178 cases and called this discrepancy "symmetrical." The left leg was more than 5 mm shorter in 32, the right one in 114. Ingelmark and Lindstrom (1963) examined 370 patients with back pain. They reported their measurements in millimeters and found differences in 87%. Shortening of the right leg was more frequently present, a fact which has been observed by other authors.

The significant increase in length of the left leg seems to be related to the higher instance of right handedness. Marsk demonstrated in 1958 that patients whose dominant hand was the right one were more prone to use the left leg as their supporting extremity while standing.

According to these investigations it is evident that leg length discrepancies are frequently observed. Lesser discrepancies require little compensation and usually do not cause difficulties. The "diagnosis" of a pelvic tilt is not uncommonly made by a tailor while fitting his customers.

2. Progression of Leg Length Discrepancies

The importance of etiological and pathogenic factors causing leg length discrepancies have been described. They alone are not sufficient to establish a proper prognosis. The reason for this is the difficulty of predicting further progression during the period of bone growth. There is no doubt that at the end of bone growth, differences in the time of closure of the epiphyseal plate can result in changes in leg length discrepancies or on occasion even cause them.

In patients suffering from poliomyelitis we were able to differentiate between rapidly progressive and nonprogressive leg length discrepancies. Stimulation of the epiphyseal plate by hyperemia in childrens' fractures lasts from 6 to 12 months. After its cessation discrepancies remain constant until puberty.

Any change in the leg length discrepancy is quite apart from those factors influencing the epiphyseal plate during the later stages of puberty. This progression of the discrepancy is of the utmost prognostic significance. In the individual patient it is therefore necessary to check leg length at regular intervals. This alone allows proper evaluation of changes of leg length discrepancies and their prognosis.

3. Clinical Observations of Leg Length Discrepancies

Most patients perceive the presence of leg length discrepancies as a marked impairment of their body integrity. They are worried that they will have to walk with a limp for the rest of their lives and are mainly concerned about the cosmetic aspects of their deformity. Leg length discrepancy results in a pelvic tilt which consequently leads to a scoliotic deformity of the spine. These changes cause asymmetry of the shape of the body which, as previously mentioned, is frequently first recognized by a dressmaker or a tailor. Leg length discrepancies of 1 to 2 cm result in a "short leg limp", which causes not only a change in the normal gait pattern but also requires additional unphysiological muscle activity. The center of gravity of the body moves normally in a rather flat sinus curve if both legs are of equal length. Short leg gait results in a marked distortion of this curve, as the center of gravity is forced to change its position on a vertical plane, resulting in an increase in energy consumption. Of greater importance than the cosmetic appearance and the relatively small increase in energy consumption are other functional disturbances caused by the pelvic tilt. It affects the spine and the hip joint and can result in serious disorders. An orthopaedist who treats a patient with a leg length discrepancy has to consider how this change will affect the patient clinically, if treatment is necessary, and what type of therapy may be required in the future.

3.1 Changes in Hip Joint Mechanics Due to Leg Length Discrepancies

Mathematical calculations by Pauwels have shown that a lesser amount of pressure is transmitted to the hip joint of the shorter leg. This occurs as a result of the pelvic tilt which increases the area of contact between the femoral head and the acetabulum. Another factor is the overhang of the body to the side of the shorter leg resulting in a shorter lever arm resulting from the lateral displacement of the center of gravity.

It is easy to demonstrate trigonometrically the increase or decrease of covering of the the femoral head by the acetabulum as a result of leg length discrepancy (Fig. 1). A distance of 25 cm between the centers of both hip joints and a shortening of one leg by 2 cm causes a decrease in covering on the longer side and an increase in covering on the shorter side. There is a reciprocal change in the C-E angle of Wiberg of approximately 4.5°.

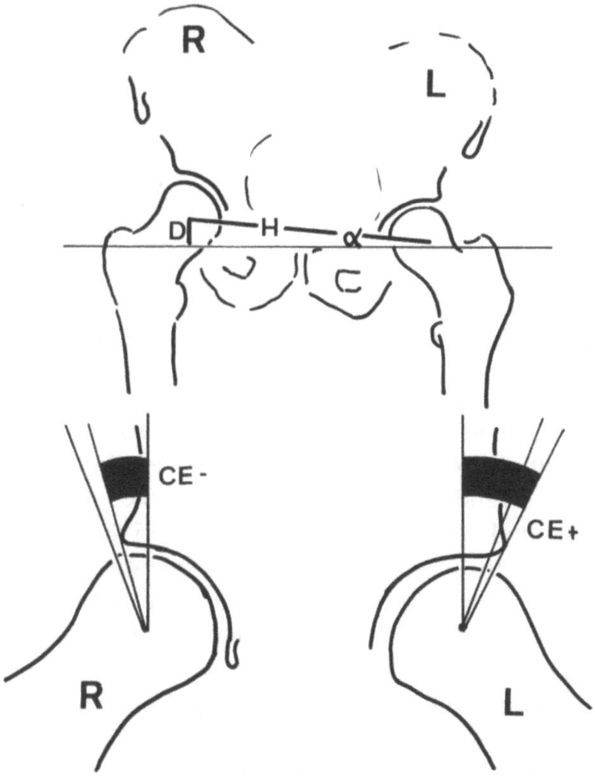

Fig. 1. Changes in C=E angle as a result of leg length discrepancies. Assuming that the difference between the two legs is 2 cm and that the distance between both centers of the hip joints is 25 cm, one gets an angle α of $4^1/_2{}^\circ$ according to the formula: sin = D/H: $^2/_{25}$ = 1.008 = $4^1/_2{}^\circ$. The femoral head of the longer leg loses the same amount of contact, the femoral head of the shorter leg gains the same amount of contact, i. e. the C=E angle is changed accordingly

The load at the hip joint of the longer leg is increased, not only by the diminution of the area of contact but also by increase in tone of the abductors as shown by Merchant (1965). The amount of diminution or enlargement of the areas of contact can be obtained from calculations by Krakovits (1972) (Table 2). Leg length discrepancies therefore act on the longer leg like a coxa valga deformity.

Increase in distance between origin and insertion of the hip abductors of the longer leg tends to increase tension of these muscles. Due to the mechanical overuse, pressure is exerted by the iliotibial tract at the greater trochanter, causing chronic trochanteric bursitis (Bopp, 1971). Nearly all of Bopp's patients with leg length discrepancies complained of pain in the trochanteric area. Four of our own 22 patients, who required a shortening osteotomy to accomplish equalization of leg length, had similar pain patterns. Bopp demonstrated further that these faulty static conditions resulted in tendinopathies at the insertion and origin of the iliopsoas at the lesser trochanter, at the transverse processes of the lumbar vertebrae and at the origin of the hip adductors, at the pubis.

Table 2. Effects of leg length discrepancies on femoral head coverage according to Krakovitz

Leg shortened by:	Diminution of C=E angle of Wiberg
1 cm	= 2.3°
2 cm	= 4.6°
3 cm	= 6.8°
4 cm	= 9.1°
5 cm	= 11.3°
6 cm	= 13.5°
7 cm	= 15.6°
8 cm	= 17.7°
9 cm	= 19.8°
10 cm	= 21.8°

3.2 Changes of Spinal Column Alignment Due to Leg Length Discrepancies

Leg length discrepancies result in pronounced changes in the spinal column, mainly in the lumbar segments. It is usually stated that the converxity of the scoliosis resulting from a pelvic tilt is directed toward the shorter leg, but this is not always the case. Ingelmark and Lindstrom (1963) found that the convexity of the lumbar scoliosis was directed toward the short side in 75% of their patients when the right side was shorter; in 87% when the left side was shorter. They found no definite correlation between pelvic tilt and the convexity of the lumbar scoliosis. They advised that one not draw conclusions from the position of the iliac crests in regard to the direction of the lumbar scoliosis. An amazingly high incidence of 34 so-called contralateral scolioses had been noted by Scheller (1964) in his 109 patients with leg length discrepancies. Beugert (1970) found contralateral scoliosis in 10% of his patients. It is quite probable that the development of a lumbar scoliosis is mainly the result of dynamic forces caused by ambulation (Leger, 1959; Taillard and Morscher, 1965), and not by static forces caused by standing.

In examining the patient it is important not only to observe the scoliosis but all other mechanisms used to overcome the leg length difference. Pelvic tilt is only one way to compensate for the discrepancy. It is effective only in differences of less than 2 cm. Larger discrepancies have to be compensated by bringing the foot into an equinus position, or even by flexing the hip and knee joint of the longer leg.

It is customary to evaluate lateral deviations of the spinal column of patients with leg length discrepancies only in the frontal plane. Yet pelvic tilt is usually combined with pelvic rotation, as demonstrated by Seidel (1969) who used four scales to demonstrate body weight distribution. This sagittal tilt results in ventral rotation of the ilium at the side of the shorter leg. The rotation, if present, may even become more pronounced if the leg length discrepancy is corrected by raising the heel of the shoe only.

Pelvic tilt as a factor in developing true scoliosis has been discussed by many authors. In general they deny this possibility. Yet there is evidence that even a small amount of pelvic tilt can result in typical changes of a true structural scoliosis, if the tilt has been present for some time and if it has not been corrected. Fixed lateral deviation, torsion of the spine on its longitudinal axis and changes in the configuration of the vertebral bodies have been observed. Scheller (1964) noted that full compensation of the deviation was possible in only 10% of his patients with leg length discrepancies. The other 90% had fixed scolioses. Wedging of vertebral bodies is to be expected only in such cases where lateral deviation of the spine originated during the period of growth.

Lateral deviations of the spine caused by pelvic tilt are in general compensated, i.e. the lumbar curve corresponds with a similar curve of the dorsal spine. Satisfactory compensation and as a result, satisfactory movement of the spinal column, influences the prognosis and probable development of back pain. It is therefore absolutely necessary in correcting leg length discrepancies to evaluate statics and dynamics of the spine thoroughly and to check the results of the correction carefully. It is difficult to improve lateral curvatures of the spinal column if spinal mobility was restricted at the time leg length was equalized (Fig. 2).

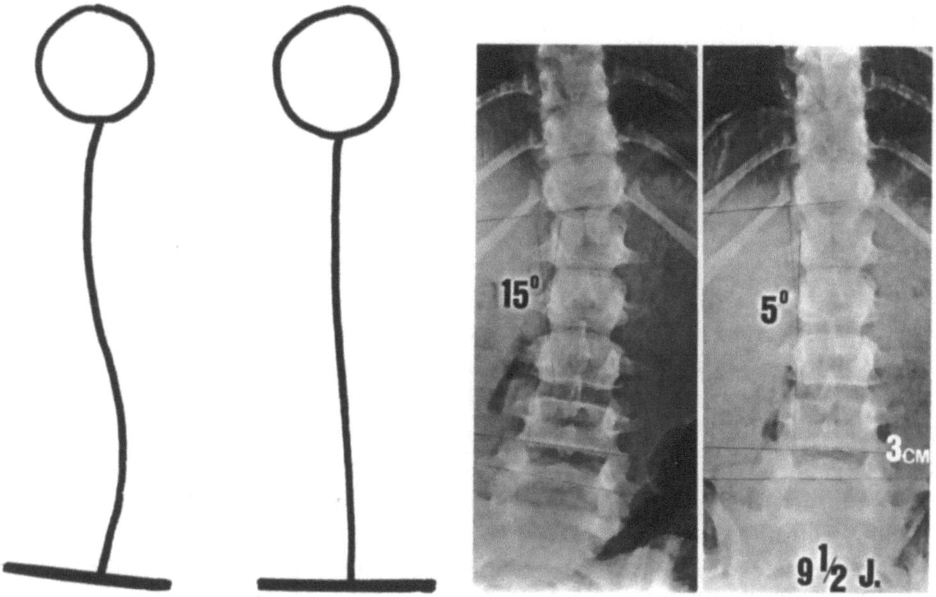

a b c d

Fig. 2. Correction of scoliosis of a flexible lumbar spine with convexity towards the site of the shorter limb. (a) and (b) Schematic drawing of effect of compensating for leg length discrepancy. (c) and (d) Boy of age $9^1/_2$ with 3 cm shortening of the lower limb. By raising the heel and the sole of the right shoe it is possible to reduce the scoliotic curve of the lumbar spine from 15 ° to 5 °

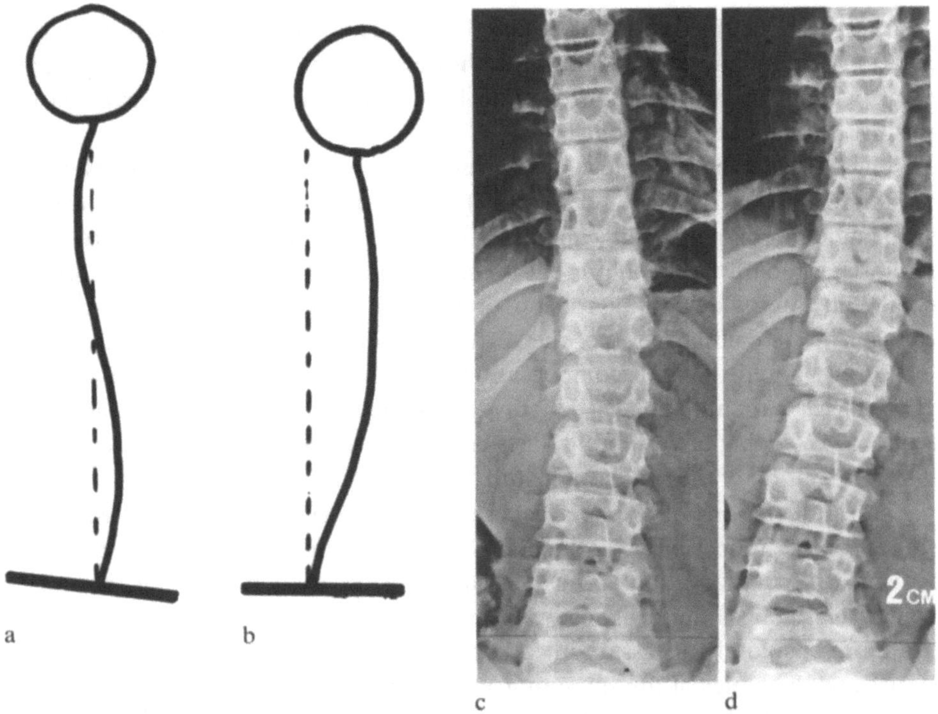

Fig. 3. Decompensation of spine due to correction of unequal lower limb length. (a) and (b) Schematic drawing demonstrating poor result of correction. Scoliotic curve is no longer compensated. (c) and (d) Lumbar scoliosis with 2 cm lower limb length discrepancy. After correction, decompensation of the scoliosis, i. e. moving of the complete spine toward the convexity of the scoliotic curve (12-year-old girl)

In the presence of a rigid fixation of the spine such correction is unlikely to achive full correction of the deformity. The result, then, of the equalization of the leg length discrepancy would be to decompensate the scoliosis, i.e., a lateral overhang of the upper part of the body (Fig. 3).

In such cases it is advisable to correct the leg length discrepancy in stages and, if necessary, with an appropriate intensive back exercise program. Particularly difficult therapeutic problems are encountered if leg length discrepancies are corrected suddenly, i.e., in shortening osteotomies. On many occasions we were astonished to note how quickly lateral spinal curvatures became fixed. On the other hand, it is difficult to correct a scoliosis even when its cause, i.e., the pelvic tilt, has been fully rectified. We therefore recommend X-ray control of every conservative or operative correction of leg length discrepancies. Functional leg length differences, asymmetric configurations of the pelvis, and malformations of the vertebral bodies can easily result in errors of interpretation.

Our own electromyographic examinations (Taillard and Morscher, 1965) have shown that relatively small leg length discrepancies of 1 to 2 cm can lead to a remarkable increase in muscle activity of several muscle groups. Even these small differences make it impossible to maintain a complete resting position.

Asymmetrical loading forces acting on the spine result in early degenerative processes affecting the intervertebral disc spaces in the form of osteochondroses, development of marked osteophyte formation on the concavity of scoliosis and an arthrosis of the facet joints. The pathogenesis of these changes is usually easily explainable (Fig. 4).

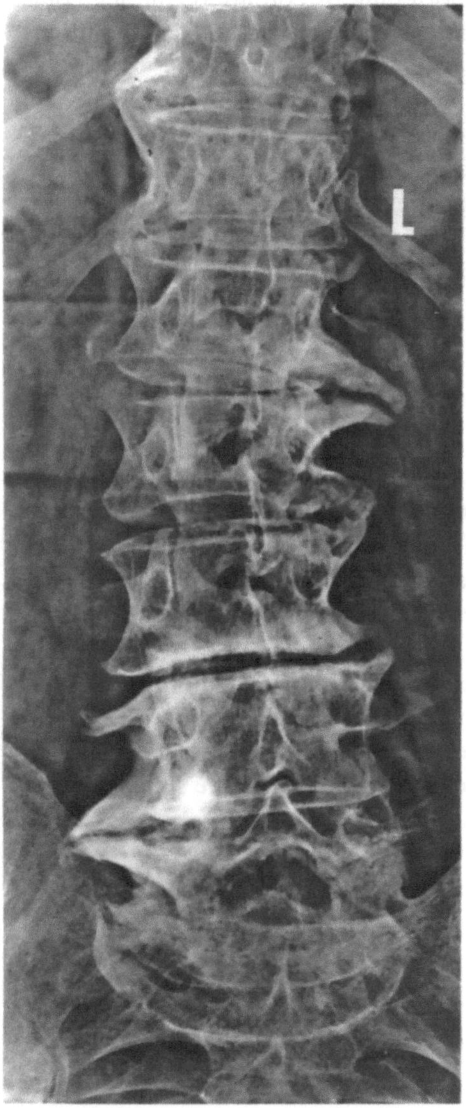

Fig. 4. Pronounced osteochondrotic and spondylotic changes of a scoliotic lumbar spine. Osteophytes are typically present on the concavity, the area of compression. Convexity of the scoliotic curve between L-1 and L-3 to the right, from L-4 to the sacrum to the left

Degenerative changes of the spinal column are frequently noted at an early stage. Yet various reports show that one should not overrate lateral spinal curvatures as a cause of backaches. Rush and Steiner (1947) reported on 100 completely healthy soldiers without any back complaints in the presence of 71 % leg length discrepancies. The same authors noted in 100 patients with backaches a leg length difference in 77%. Hult (1954) stated that 53.7% of patients with leg length discrepancies complained of lumbar pain, but 59.9% of patients without leg length discrepancies had similar complaints.

Nachemson came to a similar conclusion after examining a large group of Swedish patients with scoliosis. Wolck (1968) found no correlation between leg length discrepancies and low back pain in a group of 77 above–knee amputees. However, 19 of 50 patients who had a shortening osteotomy of the leg complained of back pain prior to surgery. Seventeen of these had no back symptoms postoperatively (Gernets, 1966).

Many publications and daily clinical experience leave no doubt that unequal leg length is a frequent cause of symptoms in the hip, pelvic or spinal areas. These functional changes may occur in the presence of differences of as little as 1 cm, as demonstrated by electromyographic examinations. It is therefore imperative to correct these discrepancies. The consequences of such a correction have to be carefully checked, as functional derangements and ailments may become aggravated by it, for instance in cases of a fixed scoliosis.

Conclusion

There are many reasons for leg length discrepancies. Idiopathic differences may amount to 2 or more centimeters and are frequently missed on examination. The prognosis of leg length discrepancy depends mainly on etiological factors. The outcome in individual cases can be predicted fairly accurately only by following the patient over many years.

Leg length discrepancies can result in esthetic or functional alterations. Static and dynamic changes of the spinal column and the hip joint are of major importance. Therefore, correction of even minor degrees of leg length differences is recommended. Their consequences, particularly in regard to the spinal column, should be carefully checked.

References

Beugert, O.: Z. Orthop. **108,** 435 (1970)
Blount, W. P.: Knochenbrüche bei Kindern. Stuttgart: G. Thieme 1957
Bopp, H. M.: Orthop. Praxis **10,** 261 (1971)
Edinger, A., Biedermann, F.: Fortschr. Röntgenstr. **86,** 754 (1957)
Ehalt, W.: Verh. dtsch. orthop. Ges. 47. Kongr. 451 (1960)
Gernet, W.: Die Verkürzungsosteotomie an den unteren Extremitäten. Inaug. Diss. 1966 (München)
Hasse, C., Dehner: Arch. Anat. Entwickl.gesch. **249,** 249 (1893)
Hult, L.: Acta orthop. scand. Suppl. 16 (1954)
Ingelmark, B. E., Lindström, J.: Acta morph. scand. **5,** 221 (1963)
König, P.: Verh. dtsch. orthop. Ges. **90,** 343 (1958)
Krakovits, G.: Statik und Dynamik des Hüftgelenkes. Z. Orthop. **102,** 418 (1967)
Leger, W.: Die Form der Wirbelsäule mit Untersuchungen über ihre Beziehungen zum Becken und die Statik der aufrechten Haltung. Stuttgart: Enke (1959)
Mac Ewen, G. D., Case, J. L.: Chir. Orthop. **50,** 147 (1967)
Marsk, A.: Acta orthop. scand. Suppl. 31 (1958)

Merchant, A. C.: J. Bone Jt Surg. **47 A,** 462 (1965)
Ratliff, A. H. C.: J. Bone Jt Surg. **47 B,** 56 (1959)
Rush, W. A., Steiner, H. A.: Amer. J. Roentgenol. **56,** 616 (1946)
Scheller, M. L.: Über den Einfluß der Beinverkürzung auf die Wirbelsäule. Inaug. Diss. Köln (1964)
Schneider, P. G.: Z. Orthop. **98,** 43 (1964)
Seidel, A.: Man. Med. **7,** 1 (1969)
Sollmann, A. H.: Orthop. **9,** 380 (1959)
Staheli, L. T.: Chir. Orthop. **55,** 159 (1967)
Taillard, W.: Verh. dtsch. orthop. Ges. 53. Kongr. 151 (1966)
Taillard, W.: Verh. dtsch. orthop. Ges. 53. Kongr. 164 (1966)
Taillard, W., Morscher, E.: Beinlängenunterschiede. Basel: Karger (1965)
Ward, J., Lerner, H.: J. Pediat. **31,** 403 (1947)
Wölck, H. J.: Funktionelle Röntgendiagnostik der Wirbelsäule bei Oberschenkelamputation. Inaug. Diss. Kiel (1968)

English translation from the German edition *Der Orthopäde,* Vol. 1, pp. 1–8 (1972),

Measurement of Leg Length

E. Morscher and G. Figner*

Measurement of leg length must be included in every examination of the lower extremities, the hip joints, or the back, especially when in the latter a lateral curvature can be confirmed. This measurement as a rule is performed clinically. Only in exceptional cases is a roentgenologic measurement necessary, e.g., when a greater degree of accuracy is required before surgical intervention, or for investigative reasons.

In these cases, to measure means to compare. One method is to measure linearly in centimeters and millimeters the distance between two points on the skeleton and, using the same measure, to compare the other extremity (direct method).

Another method for determining difference in leg length is to place boards of a known height beneath the shorter extremity until symmetry is reached. Symmetry is considered achieved when lateral pelvic obliquity and lateral spinal column curvature are corrected (indirect method).

The two methods, the direct and the indirect, are not always in accord and inasmuch as they give different values they should in all cases be used to complement each other. With the direct method, we determine the distance between two points on the skeleton and thus, essentially, the lengths of bones. With the indirect method, we get a picture of the effective total length of the lower extremity, or else the difference in length that is present in possibly existing functional differences in length caused by joint contractures, foot deformities, pelvic asymmetries, etc. In other words, correction of a difference in leg length does not follow from direct measurement of length alone but only after an "adjusting" examination has been performed. It is a scientific principle that any measurement must be reproducible. Accordingly, all measurements must follow clearly systematized and precisely defined conditions.

1. Clinical Methods of Measurement

a) Direct Measurement with the Tape Measure

With the tape measure we determine the distance between two points that are drawn on the body. Consequently, the accuracy of the measurement depends

* Orthopädische Universitätsklinik Basel, Basel, Switzerland

first of all on precise determination of these reference points. Since direct measurement is basically a question of determining bone length, one always attempts to choose points that most closely correspond to the ends of the long bones. The most difficult point to determine is the proximal end of the femur because the hip joint is not palpable due to a thick and deep surrounding layer of soft tissue. Following the advice of anthropologists (Martin, 1925, 1926) one generally uses today the anterior superior iliac spine which can always be palpated, even in obese patients. This is best performed at the tendinous origin of the sartorius, i.e., one places the tape on this tendon and pushes it with his finger cephalad against the iliac spine.

The interarticular space where the distal end of the femur and the proximal end of the tibia articulate has proved to be the best measuring point. On account of its great mobility the patella should not be used for measurements, nor should it be used as a starting point for measuring circumference.

At the distal end of the lower leg the protuberances of the medial malleolus on the inner aspect and the lateral malleolus on the outer side serve as fixed reference points.

The examiner must be familiar with the relatively great potential for error with the direct method if he is to avoid inappropriate treatment. It goes without saying, of course, that in measuring one should always use the same tape. The various tape measures on the market, mostly metal or produced from flexible material (cloth, plastic), show differences of 1–2%. This fact alone shows that the measured values are not absolute but can only be assessed comparatively. In addition to determining measuring points, which requires practice on the part of the examiner, there are, above all, functional differences that place the accuracy of the method in question. Thus a difference in the tilt of the pelvis or contractures of the hip or knee joint can considerably alter functional leg length. Not uncommonly, asymmetries in the pelvic area or asymmetric foot deformities are found in pathologic conditions of the lower extremities. One should watch especially for axial deformities of the knee joint such as genu valgum, varum, or flexum.

To determine effective thigh length one can use the distance from the anterior superior iliac spine to the lateral joint line at the knee, and for total leg length the distance from the anterior superior iliac spine to the lateral malleolus lateralis. For these measurements the tape should not be used on the medial surfaces (medial joint line, medial malleolus), because even minimal developmental asymmetry of the thigh musculature can lead to considerable error. It is not uncommon to find differences in the circumference of the thigh in the presence of leg differences (atrophy of the quadriceps muscle). Due to the larger development of the calf muscles on the outer side, if only the length of the lower leg is to be measured the distance from the medial joint line of the knee to the tip of the medial malleolus is more accurate (Fig. 1).

The degree of accuracy of the direct method is of the order of magnitude of ±0.5–1 cm.

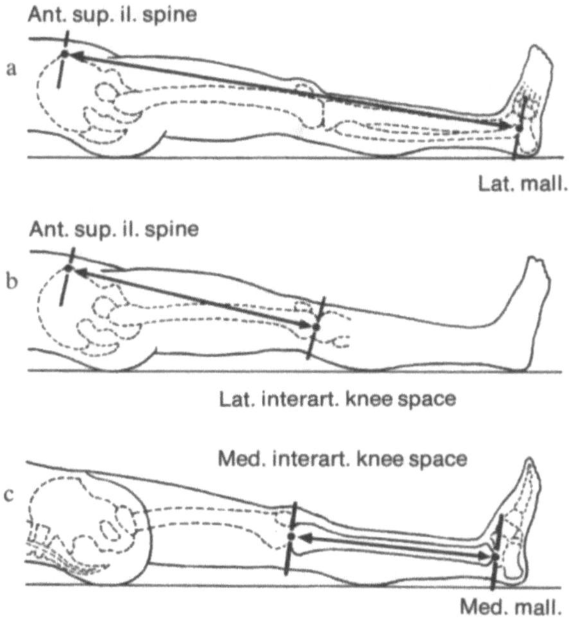

Fig. 1. Clinical measurement of leg length with the tape measure.
(a) Total leg length: anterior superior iliac spine to lateral malleolus. (b) Thigh length: anterior superior iliac spine to lateral interarticular knee space. (c) Lower leg length: medial interarticular knee space to medial malleolus (from Taillard and Morscher)

b) Indirect Methods of Measurement

Normally, the pelvis (i.e., when symmetrically formed) of a person standing erect with legs of equal length is horizontal. However, whenever the distance from the iliac crest to the base of the feet is unequal, one observes a tilt of the

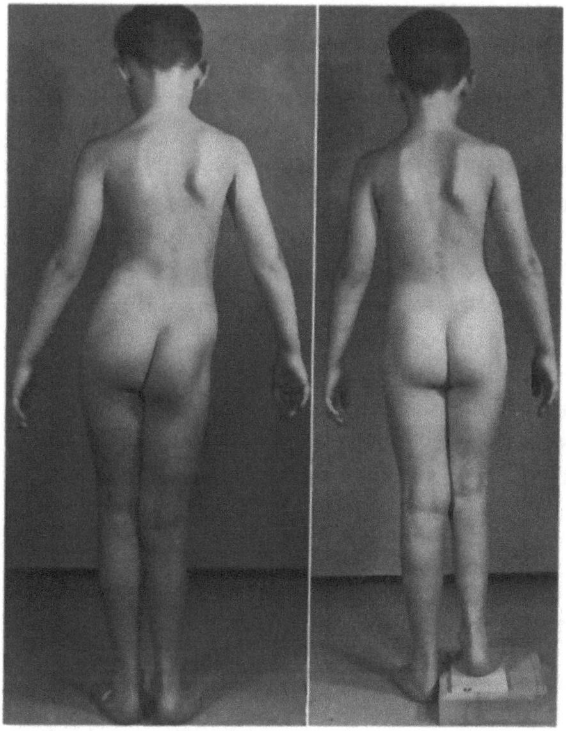

Fig. 2. Indirect measurement of leg length. The shorter leg is "built up" by placing boards of known height beneath it until the pelvis is horizontal and the lateral spinal curvature is corrected

pelvis toward the side of the shorter leg that is directly proportional to the degree of shortening. It should, of course, be borne in mind that all differences in leg length result in pelvic obliquity, but not every pelvic obliquity is caused by difference in leg length. Pelvic asymmetries, being not all that uncommon, can simulate disparities in leg length and accordingly a check of leg length by the direct method is indicated in all such cases. However, from a practical point of view, assessment of pelvis obliquity is generally quite dependable. It is in other respects independent of the cause of the shortening of the leg, i. e., independent of whether the difference in length is real or purely functional.

Measurement of leg length by means of the indirect method is carried out by placing boards of known height beneath the shorter leg until the pelvic obliquity is corrected (Fig. 2).

In cases in which the difference in leg length must be determined to the millimeter because surgical correction is planned, or on other scientific grounds, roentgenologic measurement is recommended.

2. Roentgenologic Methods of Measurement

There are basically three methods which are more or less equally accurate. They differ essentially only in technique.

2.1 **Teleradiography** (Hickey, 1924)

In teleradiography both lower extremities are filmed and measured in their entire length. In order to minimize errors arising from divergence of the path of the rays, the patient should be positioned as far as possible from the X-ray tube. Apart from that, a drawback of the method is that very large films and powerful X-ray tubes are necessary. In addition, the varying radiolucency of the leg resulting from differences in the thickness of the soft tissue layer poses difficult roentgen problems. Leger (1966) has suggested that wedge-shaped filter screens be used to compensate for this. Nevertheless, the disadvantage of this method lies in the poor contrast in the vicinity of the ankle joint (Gajewski, 1956), where finally the reference points must be measured. Another possibility of compensating for thickness consists in adapting the exposure time to the thickness of the leg (Edinger et al., 1956). Recently, experiments have been carried out with a rotating compensation diaphragm (Oest and Sieberg, 1971).

2.2 **Scanography** (Millwee, 1937)

In this method a narrow roentgen beam is moved over the distance to be measured. Here also large formats are needed in order that the bony parts may be visualized without enlargement. The great technical effort and need for large films make this method difficult to carry out.

2.3 Orthoroentgenography (Green et al., 1946; Bell and Thomson, 1950; Goldstein and Dreisinger, 1950; Taillard, 1956; Goff, 1960)

Orthoroentgenography demands the least technical expenditure with the same degree of accuracy as the methods described above. Although various modifications have been proposed, in the following we shall describe only those employed by us and suggested by Taillard in 1956 (Fig. 3). The patient lies upon a special frame on which a metal rule is placed whose calibrations are easily visible on the roentgenogram. The individual long bones need not be filmed in their entire length; simple orthogonal demonstration of the ends of the bones – the areas of the hip joint, the knee joint, and the upper ankle joint – suffice. With the patient supine, anteroposterior views are taken of the hip, knee, and ankle joints. As measuring points the upper margin of the femoral head and the lower margin of the medial femoral condyle serve for the thigh, and for the tibia the intercondylar eminence and the inferior border of the articular surface of the

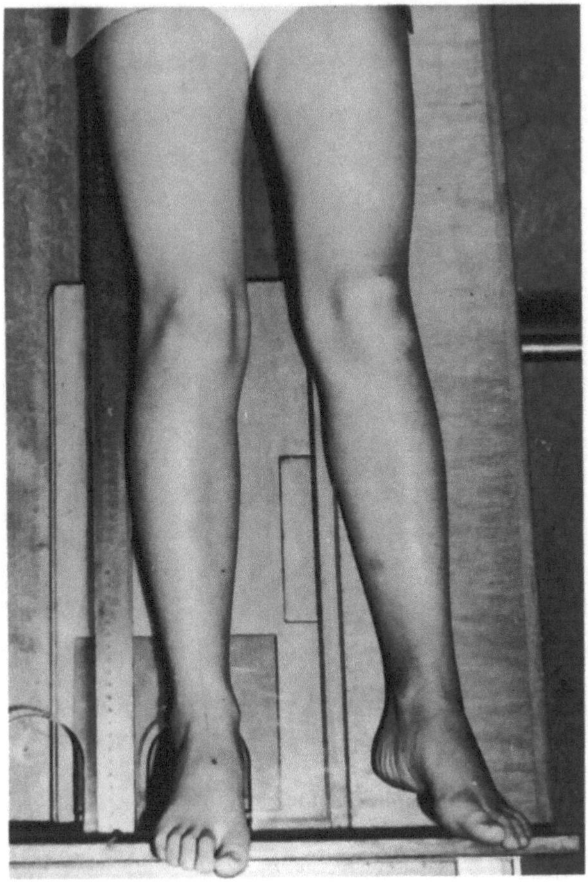

Fig. 3. Table for roentgenologic measurement of leg length (orthoroentgenography)

tibia at the ankle joint. By subtraction the lengths of the femur and tibia can then be measured accurately to the millimeter (Fig. 4).

However, orthoroentgenography is also not free of error. Such can result from inexact centering of the roentgen ray, and further, from contractures in the area of the hip or knee joints. Also the patient must not move between the various exposures.

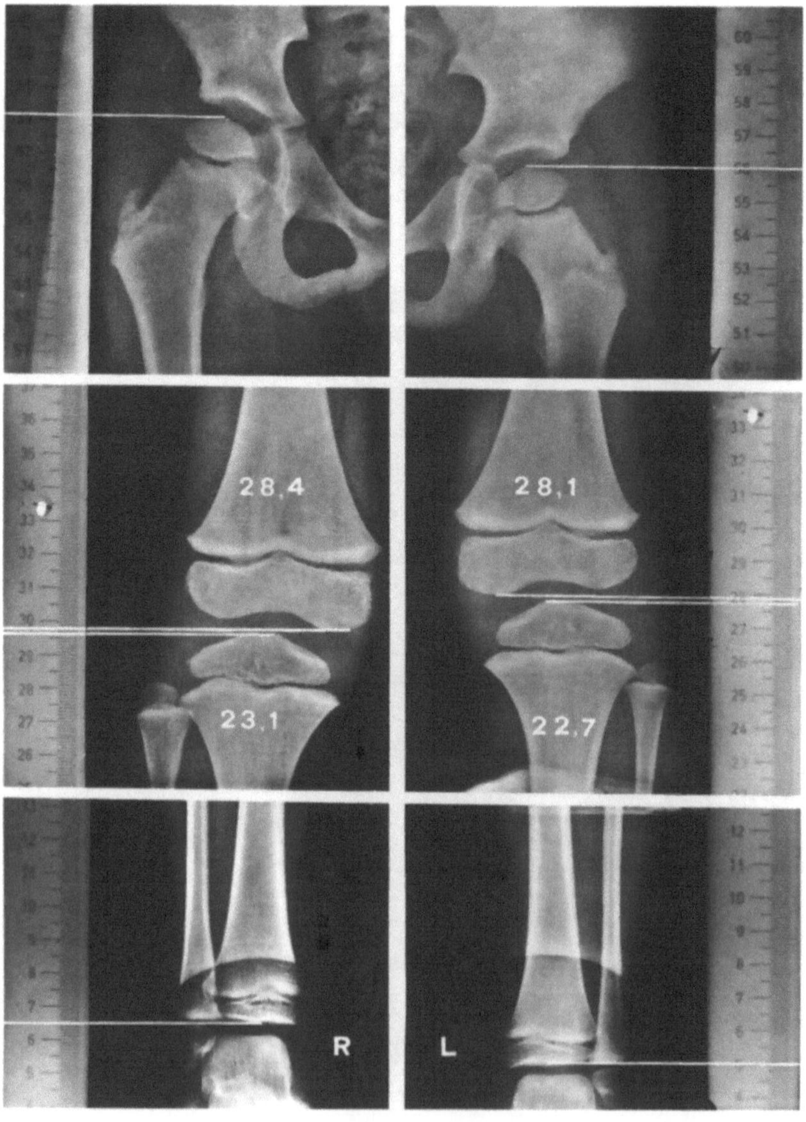

Fig. 4. So-called measuring films for exact determination of leg length

Summary

The different methods of measuring leg length are described and possible sources of error are discussed. The authors distinguish between direct and indirect methods which in every case are complementary. Their degree of accuracy lies between 0.5 and 1.0 cm. For greater accuracy in measurement, roentgenologic methods must be called upon. Among these the authors prefer orthoroentgenography.

References

Bell, J. S., Thompson, W. A. L.: Amer. J. Roentgenol. **63,** (1950)
Blount, W. P., Clarke, G. R.: J. Bone Jt Surg. **31-A,** 464 (1949)
Büchner, H.: Radiometrie. Berlin–Göttingen–Heidelberg: Springer-Verlag 1963
Edinger, A., Gajewski, H., Gepp, H.: Fortschr. Röntgenstr. **84,** 356–371 (1956)
Gajewski, H.: Röntgen-Lab. Praxis **9,** 17–30 (1956)
Goff, C. W.: Surgical Treatment of Unequal Extremities. Springfield, Ill.: Ch. C. Thomas 1960
Goldstein, L. A., Dreisinger, F.: J. Bone Jt Surg. **32-A,** 449 (1950)
Green, W. T., Wyatt, G. M., Anderson, M.: J. Bone Jt Surg. **28,** 60 (1946)
Hickey, P. M.: Amer. J. Roentgenolog. II, 232 (1924)
Leger, W.: Z. Orthop. **92,** 293 (1960)
Martin, R.: Lehrbuch der Anthropologie. Stuttgart: Fischer 1956
Millwee, R. H.: Radiol. **28,** 483 (1937)
Oest, O., Sieberg, H. J.: Z. Orthop. **109 I,** 54 (1971)
Taillard, W.: Z. Orthop. **88,** 151 (1956)
Taillard, W., Morscher, E.: Die Beinlängenunterschiede. Basel, New York: S. Karger 1965

English translation from the German edition *Der Orthopäde,* Vol. 1, pp. 9–13 (1972),

Methodological Errors in Documenting Leg Length and Leg Length Discrepancies

J. Eichler*

Varying degrees of leg length discrepancies are frequently observed during a general orthopaedic examination. We are particularly interested in quantifying the difference between the right and left legs if inequality has been noted.

Difficulties in accurately measuring these changes have resulted in many terms to describe leg length. They are defined as follows:

1. Absolute Length

Distance between the most proximal part of the femoral head and the point of contact of the foot with the ground. The contact point can be the sole of the foot, the transverse arch, the toes, or the tips of the toes.

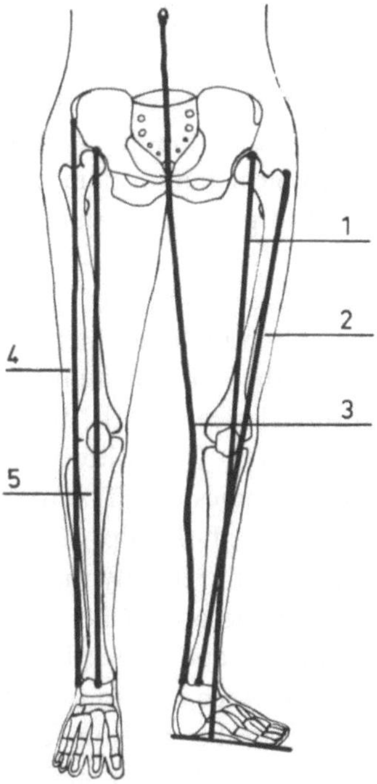

Fig. 1. Types of leg lengths. *1.* Absolute leg length. *2.* Anatomical leg length. *3.* Apparent leg length. *4.* Clinical leg length. *5.* Relative leg length

* Orthopädische Universitäts-Klinik Giessen (Director: Dr. H. Rettig), Federal Republic of Germany

2. Anatomical Length

Distance between the proximal end of the greater trochanter and the distal end of the lateral malleolus.

3. Apparent Length

Distance between umbilicus and distal end of the medial malleolus.

4. Clinical Length

Distance between anterior superior iliac spine and distal end of the lateral malleolus.

5. Functional Length

Leg shortening or lengthening caused by joint contractures or by axial malalignment.

6. Relative Length

Distance between articular surface of the hip joint and the tibio-talar joint recorded by radiographic measurement.

Absolute leg length is of relatively little importance to the practicing orthopaedist. It can only be obtained radiologically with the patient standing and it requires synchronous projection of a metal ruler. Anatomical length data are rather unreliable as it is difficult to palpate the tip of the greater trochanter accurately.

Measurements of extremities can only be carried out in the presence of well-defined landmarks. They should be easily palpable to enable other examiners to find them without difficulty. In 1925 Martin recommended the anterior superior iliac spine as the proximal point of reference for measuring clinical length; distal end points are the tip of the lateral or medial malleolus. The Committee for Documentation of the DGOT (German Society of Orthopaedics and Traumatology) in conformity with S.I.C.O.T. recommends the use of the tip of the lateral malleolus as the distal landmark for clinical length. Until recently the tip of the medial malleolus has been commonly employed as an end point (Debrunner, 1966). Measuring in this manner requires the measuring tape to be placed diagonally across the leg, introducing the shape of the leg surface as a source of inaccuracy. The distance to be measured corresponds in general to the long axis of the leg, if the lateral malleolus is the end point. This results in a slightly shorter distance in the presence of a genu valgum and a slightly longer distance in the presence of a genu varum (Fig. 2.)

It is advisable to employ the iliac crest as a point of origin if the anterior superior iliac spine is absent. Measurement between umbilicus and the tip of the medial malleolus (apparent lower limb length) is not recommended as the position of the umbilicus is inconstant.

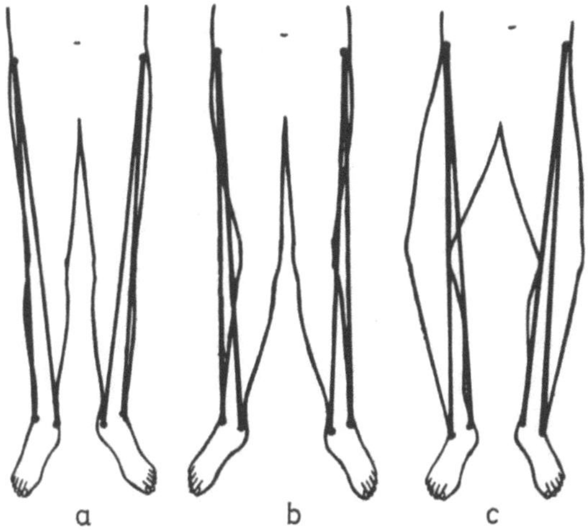

Fig. 2. (a) The distance anterior superior iliac spine to tip of lateral malleolus represents a true value in the presence of normal axial alignment of the leg. The diagonal distance to the medial malleolus does not correspond with the limb axis. (b) Genu valgum results in a shortened distance. (c) Considerable genu varum is difficult to measure, as longer distances are obtained if the tape measure follows the contour of the limb closely

I. Direct Leg Length Measurements

We suggest using a 2 cm wide tape measure made of cloth and covered by plastic material. Its zero point and scale have to be readily discernible. Metal tapes have several disadvantages. They are smaller in width, have sharper edges, do not conform readily to the contour of the leg and are annoying to patients because they feel cold. The patient should be supine on a firm examining table. His position should correspond to the neutral zero position. The tape measure should be stretched firmly between both end points and it should be placed in as straight a line as possible (Chapchal, 1971).

Measurements should be rounded off to the nearest 0.5 cm. Debrunner (1968) recommends the use of millimeter recordings to diminish measuring errors as much as possible. His calculations have shown that the mean value of range of error is between 2.4 and 3.9 mm if a millimeter scale is used. This range of error increases to 5.3 and 8.2 mm if distances are recorded in 0.5 mm gradations. According to our analysis of possible error, it suffices to record leg length differences in units of 0.5 cm, as inaccuracies are not caused by incorrect readings but by the measuring process itself.

Twenty-five persons were examined by 10 physicians and 7 medical students to evaluate methodological errors in documenting clinical leg lengths. The same tape was used by all, none knew the correct lower limb length prior to the examination. The examiners were asked to record their values in writing and not to communicate with one another. The obtained data showed a surprisingly large variability (Tables 1 and 2).

Table 1. Leg length measurements – 25 patients, leg length equal

Examiner		10 Physicians	7 Students
Maximum differences	D	4.5 cm	5.5 cm
Standard deviation	s	1.5 cm	2.5 cm
Range of error (%)	VK	1.9%	2.3%

Table 2. Leg length measurements – 10 patients, leg length different

Examiner		10 Physicians	
Segment measured		Rt. leg	Lt. leg
Maximum difference	D	5.0 cm	4.9 cm
Standard deviation	s	2.0 cm	2.0 cm
Range of error	VK	2.1%	2.1%

Additional examinations of several patients, using full length leg X-rays, were carried out and evaluated. Radiological examination measures relative leg length only. Therefore it was impossible to correlate these findings with the clinical observations. Differences between results obtained clinically and radiologically showed no mathematical correlation.

The analysis of clinical leg length measurement revealed the following reasons for errors:

1. Difference in Circumference of the Legs

As the tape measure is applied parallel to the leg, it documents circumferential leg size indirectly. The distance between anterior superior iliac spine and lateral

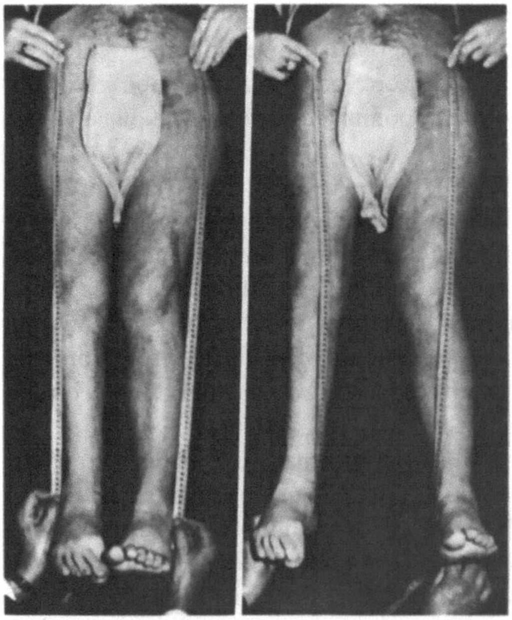

a b

Fig. 3. Male 31 years old, Poliomyelitis at age 19. Atrophy of the right leg, no leg length discrepancy. (a) Clinical leg length measurements to the tip of the lateral malleolus: right 87 cm, left 89 cm. (b) Clinical leg length measurements to the tip of the medial malleolus: right 87 cm, left 90 cm. Atrophic changes are responsible for a diminution in distance of 2 cm (lateral malleolus) and 3 cm (medial malleolus)

malleolus depends on the circumferential leg size; slimmer legs decrease the distance (Fig. 3.)

2. Unilateral Deviations of the Long Axis of the Leg

Genu valgum deformities result in measurements which are actually shorter than the real length of the leg. This is caused by the straight course of the tape measure. Genu varum deformities necessitate measuring an arc resulting in a measurement which is longer than real leg length.

3. Difficulties in Localizing the Anterior Superior Iliac Spine

Only the most anterior point of the superior iliac spine, the origin of the sartorius and tensor fasciae lata muscle, should be employed. Debrunner (1971) recommended palpating the tendons of these muscles and to trace them to their origin. Even slight obesity can create difficulties in properly localizing the anterior superior iliac spine.

4. Localization of the End Point at the Lateral Malleolus

Different examiners used different end points at the lateral malleolus. The end of the tip of the lateral malleolus, not its most lateral part, should be used as the correct end point.

5. "Pelvic Defects"

Increase in ventral inclination of the pelvis results in a decrease in clinical leg length. Pelvic asymmetry results in a difference in the position of the anterior superior iliac spine.

6. Joint Contractures

It is extremely difficult to measure clinical leg length accurately if hip joint contractures or anklyoses are present. In these cases we have to be satisfied with approximate values.

Our evaluation has shown that measurements of clinical leg lengths are fraught with methodological errors. Tape measurements of patient with healthy legs, even in the hand of experienced examiners, contain a range of error of 1.5 cm. The mean methodological range of error rises to 2 cm, if different leg lengths have to be recorded. The reason for such an increase is the presence of differences in leg circumference and joint contractures. It is therefore impossible to plan lengthening or shortening osteotomies on the basis of tape measurements

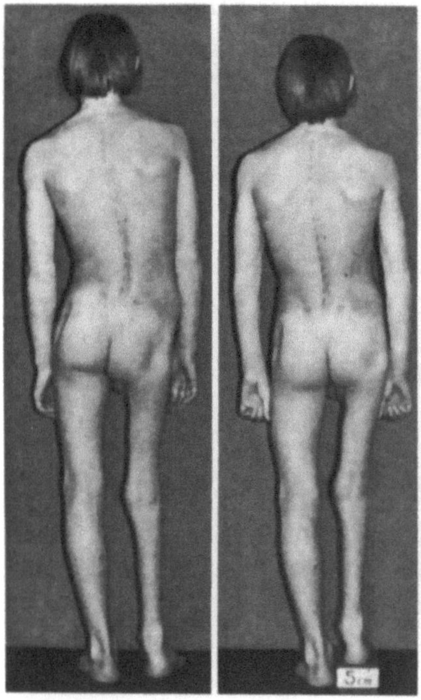

a

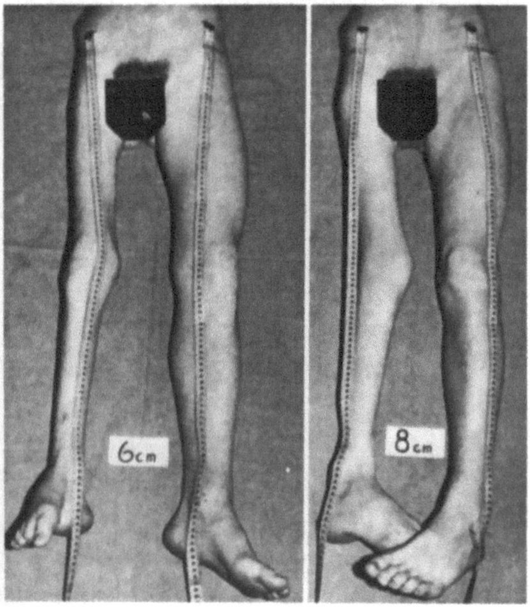

b

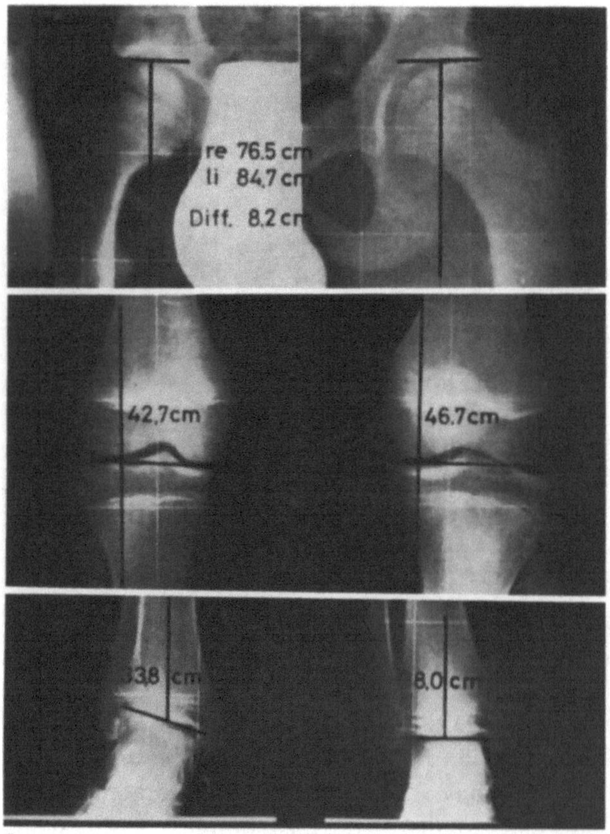

c

Fig. 4. Male 15 years old, Poliomyelitis at age 3. (a) Correction of 5 cm results in anal cleft being approximately vertical, a level pelvis and a nearly complete correction of the scoliosis. (b) Measurements of clinical leg length, to medial malleolus: 6 cm difference, to lateral malleolus, 8 cm difference. (c) Teleradiography of the same patient demonstrates a difference of 8.2 cm. This value is explained by a projection error of 6.6 %. Correction of this error results in a difference of 6 cm. Due to the presence of a malaligned axis of the right talar joint it is probable that the leg length measurement obtained by using a wooden board is correct only. This fact applies also in determining the amount of permanent disability in medico-legal cases. According to the B.V.G. (German Federal Law of Assistance), a loss of up to 3 cm of leg length does not entitle a patient to any compensation. A 20% value of permanent disability has to be awarded if one leg is shortened by 4 cm. Therefore it is unadvisable to employ a method with a 2 cm mean factor of error in evaluating borderline situations.

II. Indirect Leg Length Measurements

We measure leg length differences with wooden boards to build up the short side. With boards of 0.5, 1, 2, 3, and 5 cm thickness it is possible to document differences up to 10 cm. Measurements have to be carried out with the patient completely undressed. It is extremely important to judge conditions of leg length discrepancies not only by comparing the pelvic crests but also by observing the anal cleft, which should be in true vertical alignment. It is also important to observe sagittal deviations of the pelvis and the configuration of the spine. The examination of 10 patients without joint contractures with different leg lengths using wooden boards to equalize the discrepancy resulted in approximately similar findings to values obtained by radiographic measurements. Differences of less than 0.5 cm were noted between the two methods but they were felt to be negligible.

Documentation of leg length discrepancy is difficult if a hip joint contracture and ankylosis is present (Fig. 5). An adduction contracture of the hip joint

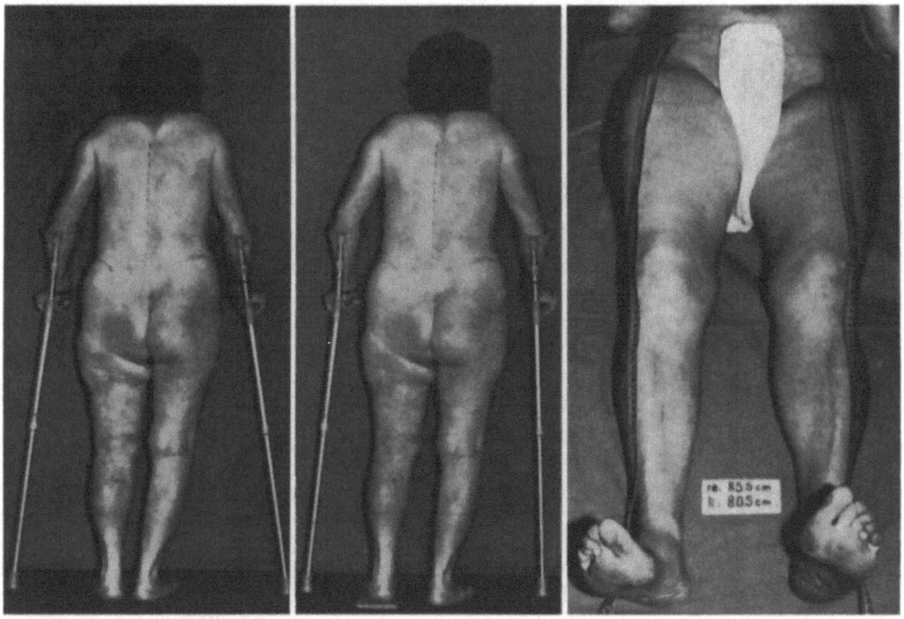

a b c

Fig. 5

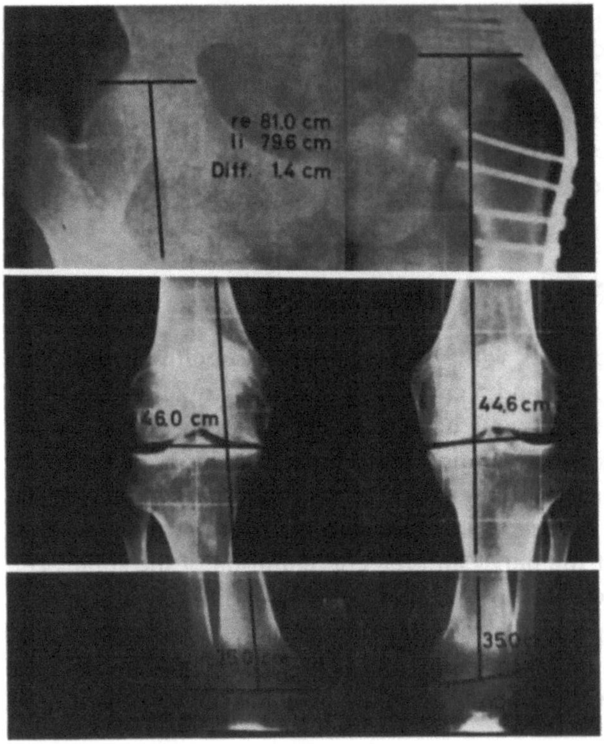

Fig. 5 d

Fig. 5. Female 53 years old. Arthrodesis of left hip, 3 weeks after surgery. (a) Standing without correction of leg length discrepancy. (b) Correction of left leg length discrepancy by 1 cm results in the patient feeling "well." Position of anal cleft cannot be properly evaluated due to obesity and atrophy of gluteal musculature. (c) Left leg length apparently 5 cm shorter by clinical leg length measurement, due to muscle atrophy, slight genu valgum and a hip flexion contracture of 20%. (d) Radiographic limb measurement difference 1.4 cm

results in functional shortening of the involved lower limb. This can be corrected by raising the right side of the pelvis. Our example (Fig. 6) shows the pelvic crest on the side of the contracture to be 4 cm higher than the other crest, but 6 cm wooden board correction is required to have the patient put an equal amount of

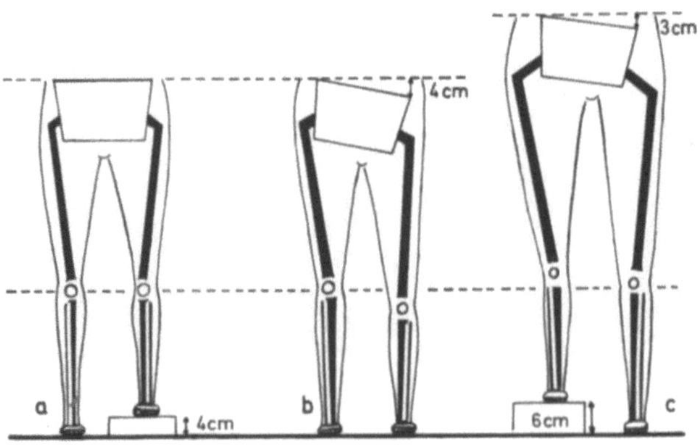

Fig. 6. (a) One leg 4 cm shorter, corrected by wooden boards. (b) Ilium tilts 4 cm downward after removal of the wooden boards: true anatomical shortening of the leg. (c) Adduction contracture of one hip: 6 cm wooden board correction required due to the presence of 3 cm functional and 3 cm anatomical leg length discrepancy

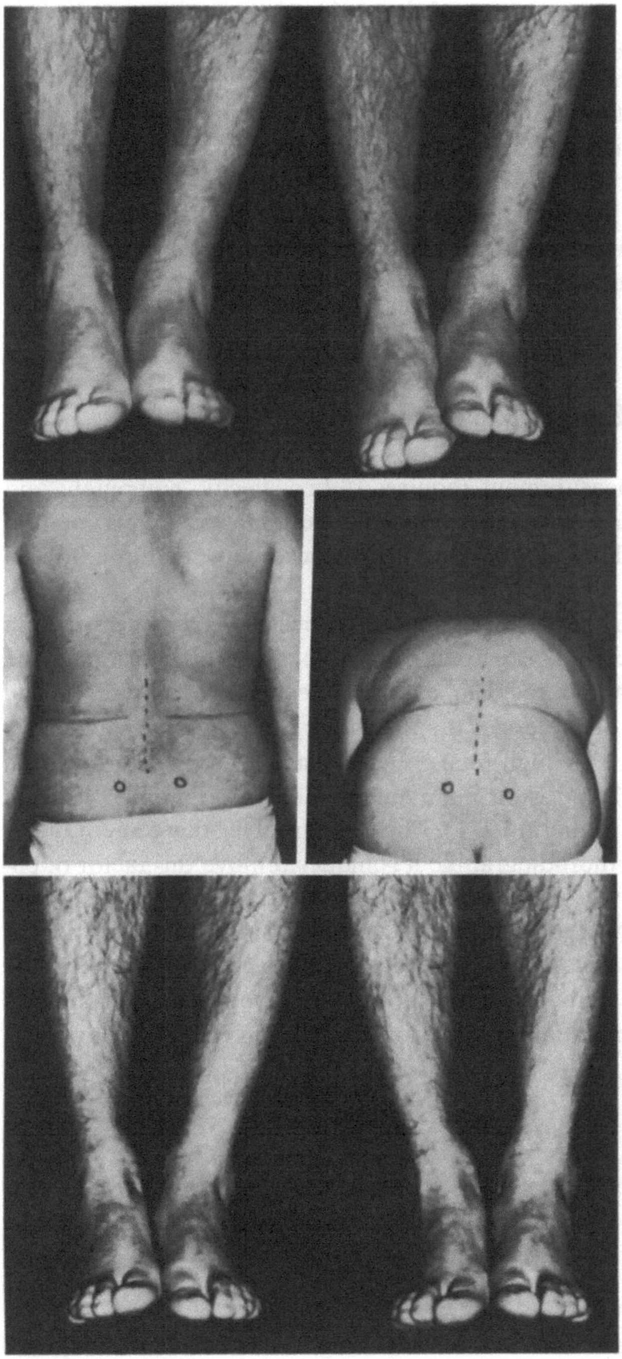

a

b

c

Fig. 7. Male 24 years old, "blocked" left sacroiliac joint. (a) Left side: leg length with the patient supine, neutral zero position. Right side: leg length sitting, left leg 1.5 cm shorter. (b) Iliac crests essentially level. Flexion of the lumbar spine results in a cephelad displacement of the left posterior iliac spine. (c) After "manipulation" of the left sacroiliac joint, leg length equal with patient supine (left side) and sitting (right side)

weight on the soles of both feet. The difference is explained by the presence of a functional discrepancy of 4 cm and a real discrepancy of 2 cm.

It is even more difficult to evaluate leg length discrepancies in patients with fusions of the hip joint, asymmetry of the pelvis and scoliosis. In these cases one has to rely on the subjective statements of the patient in regard to satisfactory correction. Examining the patient in a supine position with shoes being worn by him allows one to estimate if an addition to the sole of his shoe is necessary.

Leg length measurements with the patient supine or sitting may show small lower limb differences which are dependent on the particular position of the patient. They can alert us to the presence of a blocked sacroiliac joint if a change in position of the posterior iliac spine during flexion of the lumbar spine is noted at the same time. These minimal changes disappear after a vertebral manipulation. It is rarely possible to demonstrate them objectively (Fig. 7).

III. Radiographic Leg Length Measurements

Radiographic leg length measurement requires rather specific equipment and therefore is rarely used in everyday orthopaedic examinations. This method evaluates relative leg length by determining the distance between hip joint and tibio-talar joint only.

By employing teleradiography it is possible to reduce the error of projection by lengthening the distance between focus and object and by shortening the distance between object and film. The exposure techniques require special rotation diaphragms as the diameters of the tibio-talar, knee and hip joints have a relation of 1 to 1.2 to 2.3. A high focus-object distance of 3 meters and an object-film distance of 15.5 cm results in an enlargement of a femur of 40.6 cm length by 2.7 cm (Oest and Sieberg, 1971). The radiographic enlargement factor is therefore 6.6 %. Only orthoradiographic techniques remove this factor of enlargement nearly completely (Morscher and Taillard, 1965). Leg length measurements by this method require three exposures. Since the metal ruler is built into the X-ray table, it cannot be placed parallel to the lower limb in the coronal plane of the lower limb. Therefore projection errors remain in spite of the sophisticated X-ray equipment required for this method. They are, however, quite small.

Summary

The selection of a practical method for leg length measurements depends entirely on its simplicity,, exactness and ready availability. Our evaluation of different types of examination have shown that only the indirect method of leg length measurements by using wooden boards fulfills these prerequisites. The other methods require either sophisticated technical equipment or are fraught with large methodological errors.

References

Chapchal, G.: Die Untersuchung des Bewegungssystems. Handbuch der Orthopädie. Vol. I, pp. 792–827, Stuttgart: Thieme 1957
Chapchal, G., Dolanc, B., Jani, L.: Orthopädische Krankenuntersuchung. 2nd ed. Stuttgart: Enke 1971
Debrunner, H. U.: Orthopädisches Diagnostikum. Stuttgart: Thieme 1966
Debrunner, H. U.: Verh. dtsch. orthop. Ges., 54. Kongr.: 341–350 (1968)
Debrunner, H. U.: A–O Bulletin, April 1971
Martin, R.: Anthropometrie, Berlin 1925
Morscher, E., Taillard, W.: Beinlängenunterschiede. Basel. New York: S. Karger 1965
Oest, O., Sieberg, H. J.: Z. orthop. **109,** 54–72 (1971)1

English translation from the German edition *Der Orthopäde,* Vol. 1, pp. 14–20 (1972),

Equalization of Leg Length with Orthopaedic Shoe Measures

E. Meyer and D. Petersen*

I. Indications and Technical Problems

1. Introduction

In the conservative management of patients with differences in leg length, two generally well-known methods are at our disposal. Where the difference in leg length is no greater than about 2.5 cm, this relatively slight imbalance can be easily corrected by simply elevating the heel or the heel and the sole. Where the difference is between 1.5 and 2.5 cm a better cosmetic result is obtained, provided the toe-piece is sufficiently high, by fitting a 0.5–1.0 cork instep into the shoe. The goal, even in slightly shortened legs, is full equalization and balance in order to avoid static stress on the spinal column. However, with differences of over 2.5 cm, the conversion of ready-made shoes in most cases no longer suffices. Here orthopaedic shoes must be prescribed in which the correction is built into the shoe and thus becomes a fixed part of the shoe (Fig. 1). This technique is well-known and will not be discussed in detail here. Its disadvantages are equally

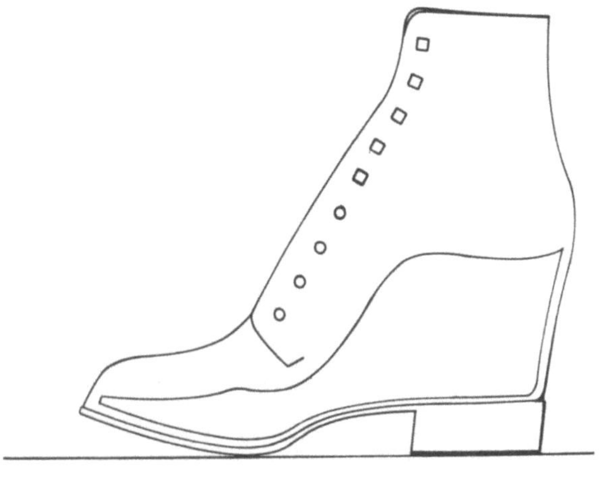

Fig. 1. Orthopaedic shoe with built-in correction (construction drawing)

* Orthopädische Heil- und Lehranstalt Annastift, Hanover-Kleefeld, Abteilung Orthopädische Schuh- und Lehrwerkstatt (Medical Director: Prof. Dr. med. G. Hauberg), Federal Republic of Germany

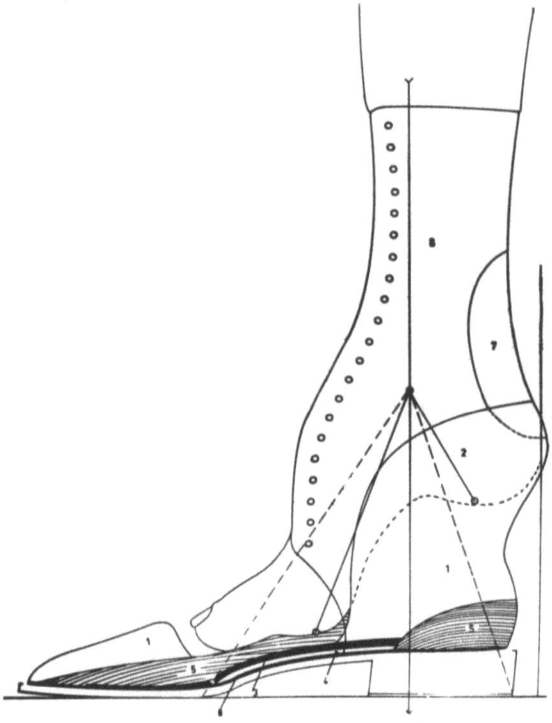

Fig. 2. Inner shoe for correction of leg length discrepancy (construction drawing)

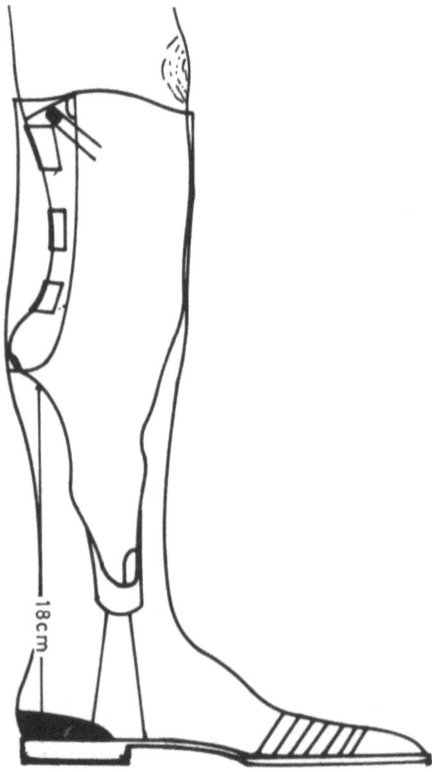

Fig. 3. Leg lengthening prosthesis (construction drawing)

well-known, both with respect to function and the cosmetic aspect. Even though complete equalization is achieved, in the case of more marked length differences the shoe becomes increasingly clumsy, heavy, and unattractive. One often hesitates to carry out this albeit necessary procedure, preferring rather to put up with the abnormal strain on the spine and on the joints of the lower extremities.

Possibly not so well-known is the use of recently designed inner shoes, in particular those utilizing the rigid foam casting resin technique. These shoes may be used in slight and moderate (Fig. 2) as well as in more extreme cases (Fig. 3). Here we are really speaking of leg lengthening prostheses. Their great advantage lies in the fact that in the majority of cases ready-made shoes can be worn.

The development of new methods at the research institute for orthopaedic shoe handicrafts at Annastift, Hannover-Kleefeld, has resulted in substantial improvements in the construction of orthopaedic inner shoes – in their function, hygiene, and cosmetic appearance. Especially favored by women and younger patients, their use is gaining considerable ground today. It goes without saying that before resorting to inner shoes, all possiblities of surgical correction should be exhausted. Surgery, however, has its limits, and in most cases inner shoes provide a satisfactory result, both in terms of function and masking the impairment. The latter consideration – the cosmetic aspect – has recently become increasingly important. Shoes are subject to frequent changes in fashion. After one or two years the patient assigned to orthopaedic shoes is faced with the possibility of having to change styles to meet the various needs of day-to-day living. The expense involved here is prohibitive. For this reason alone, many handicapped persons prefer the inner shoe because it enables them to wear ready-made shoes and, like the nonhandicapped, adapt quickly to the vagaries of fashion.

In providing patients with inner shoes, it is rarely a question of merely correcting the difference in leg length. In most cases, measures must be taken at the same time to equalize foot length, correct faulty posture, form a base for foot malpositioning, relieve the stress on pressure-sensitive areas, and provide walking aids (functional assistance). Accordingly, the inner shoe should be viewed as an orthopaedic expedient, not a shoe in the strict sense of the word, but rather an auxiliary resource that requires in addition a ready-made shoe, or even, in the exceptional case, an orthopaedically measured shoe.

With regard to the various structural features, which are determined by both the clinical picture and the applicability of the ready-made shoe, the following classification has proved useful in practice:

a) Inner shoes for shortened legs of ~ 2.5 cm (Fig. 4). As mentioned above, with leg length differences of about 2–2.5 cm, conversion of ready-made shoes is the most practicable method. With greater differences, inner shoes enter the picture. Figure 4 shows such an inner shoe correction. The material used here was rigid foam casting resin, so that hygienic considerations are adequately taken into account. By putting on a stocking over the inner shoe, the defect can be almost completely camouflaged. In almost all cases, ready-made shoes may be worn. If necessary, foot corrections, relief of pressure-sensitive areas, walking assistance, adjustments of differences in foot length, can be carried out without difficulty.

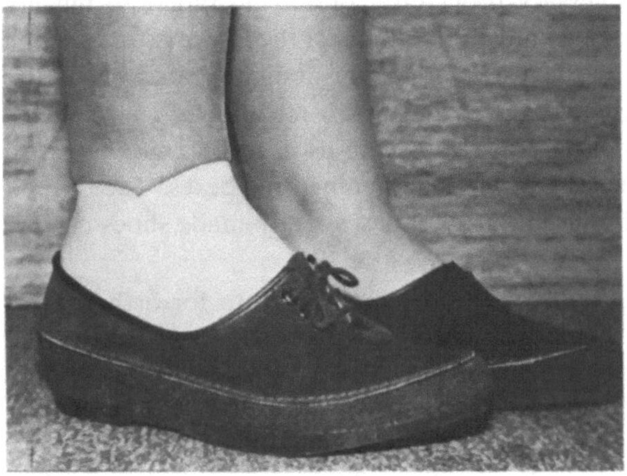

Fig. 4. Inner shoe in a discrepancy of 4 cm

b) Inner shoes for shortened legs of 6–13 cm: In shortenings of this magnitude that cannot be reduced surgically, the use of the usual orthopaedic footwear with built-in adjustments is, especially in female patients, very questionable. As a rule, in such cases, if complete balance were to be achieved in order to avoid the previously mentioned spinal stress, as well as strain on the joints of the lower extremities, the resulting orthopaedic shoe would be too heavy and clumsy, and thus the functional outcome unsatisfactory. Cosmetically, the result would be considered poor. Here the use of inner shoes creates markedly better conditions, as is demonstrated by its construction illustrated in Figure 2. Moreover, it allows for adjustments in foot length to be made without difficulty, and, of course, for any measures for relief of pressure-sensitive areas, should such become necessary. Any functional aids that are needed are installed beforehand. Wearing of ready-made shoes is usually possible; only in exceptional cases do extreme malpositions of the foot prevent this. However, all possible attempts should be made to better the condition by operative measures in order that the foot may be properly placed in the inner shoe, thus enabling the wearing of ready-made shoes.

c) Inner shoes or leg lengthening prostheses in shortened legs of 14–30 cm:

Figure 3 shows the general principles of construction. Of decisive importance in these prostheses is to bring the foot into a marked equinus (drop foot) position. Only then can a cosmetically unobjectionable result be achieved. If this cannot be managed, then the necessary conditions must be created by surgery. It is recommended, however, that, as far as possible, amputation be avoided. Even in its equinus position, the foot can serve as an intrinsically functional lengthening of the shortened leg and make a decided contribution to improved performance of the prosthesis. In the event that a partial amputation of the forefoot cannot be avoided, the plantar skin beneath the heel should be preserved in order to secure full weight bearing. It is precisely on this point that a critical distinction is made in comparison to the below-knee prosthesis. In the latter, the body weight is supported essentially by the skeletal parts, and only in a relatively small percentage of cases does it allow stable full weight-bearing by the stump. The use of ready-made shoes with the leg-lengthening prosthesis is basically no problem. The prostheses ends in a prosthetic foot of a suitable size over which the desired stocking and ready-made shoe may be worn.

2. Basic Structural Features

In the above three groups a–c with leg shortenings of approx. 2–5 cm, 6–13 cm, and 14–30 cm, respectively, there are special construction features to which attention should be called. These will be discussed individually.

Group a (2–5 cm discrepancy)

Firstly, it is important to point out that in shortened legs of this magnitude there is a frequent possibility of the prosthesis terminating below the malleolar axis. This, then, eliminates the possibility of interference with malleolar movement during walking and allows a normal "rolling off" of the foot during gait. This appears to us to be an important functional advantage. Obviously, a second stocking may be worn over the inner shoe (omitted in Fig. 4 in order to show the prosthesis). The additional stocking will provide an almost complete cosmetic masking of the device.

This means of care has its limitations with regard to conforming the prosthesis to the heel. In the length discrepancies under discussion here, the heel in every case remains within the ready-made shoe. An expedient such as that shown in Figure 5 is cosmetically unsatisfactory, especially in the case of women, because the heel protruding over the ready-made shoe will greatly impair the cosmetic appearance. This is not as important a consideration in male patients inasmuch as a long stocking will cover the protruding heel.

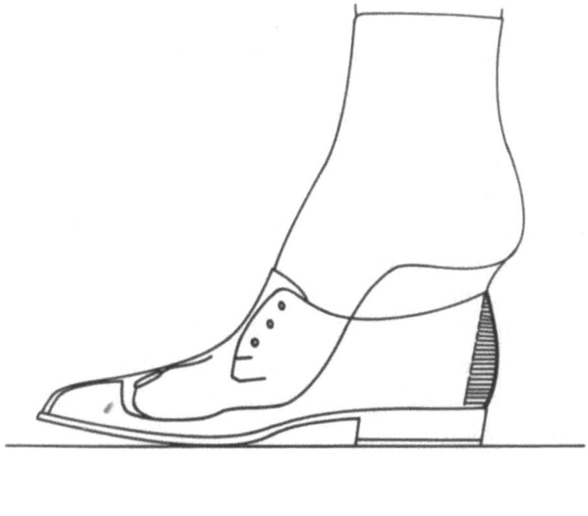

Fig. 5. Cosmetically unsatisfactory attempt to correct a moderate discrepancy

A bridge to transfer the weight of the forefoot onto the ball of the foot (Fig. 2, *3*) may be dispensed with in this group of patients since in such small differences the ball of the forefoot coincides more or less with the ball of the ready-made shoe. Since the fabrication of inner shoes poses no technical difficulties and in view of the considerable functional and cosmetic advantages over the usual orthopaedic shoes, increasing numbers of our patients prefer this method of correction.

Group b (6–13 cm discrepancy)

In this group there is no longer a possibility of the shaft of the prosthesis terminating beneath the malleoli. A higher shaft is necessary to attain at least a measure of stabilization of the ankle joint and a firm stabilization of the talocalcaneal-navicular joint. Since the latter is a number of centimeters from the ground, seesaw movements must be eliminated without fail in order to guarantee adequate security while standing and walking. Moreover, it must be borne in mind that patients with shortened legs of this magnitude are frequently inclined to tip the foot medially or laterally, depending on the malposition of the foot or leg, respectively, – defects which are difficult to correct surgically or whose operative correction is refused by the patient. This is especially the case in paralysis with loss of muscular control of the hind foot. Here, if the possibility exists to procure stability by arthrodesis, inner shoe care will be technically facilitated. If stable conditions are not present, the patient's safety is secured by readjusting the balance and providing an additional ankle support in the shaft that will bridge the talocalcaneal navicular joint. Such measures are absolutely necessary; otherwise the patient may lose his footing on an uneven surface, particularly if it is dark and he is unfamiliar with the terrain. It is important that a strong bridge be installed, one that is capable of transferring the weight of the forefoot onto the ball of the ready-made shoe, as is illustrated by *3* in Figure 2.

It may be further noted in Figure 2 that with an increase in the drop of the foot, the ball of the foot draws nearer to the long axis of the lower leg. The weight of the body, which is exerted on the forefoot, is now borne by the "shoe joint," i. e., the area of the shoe between the heel and the five metatarsal condyles upon which the foot is set down in walking. Since in ready-made shoes this area is too unstable to bear weight, the inner shoe will require a so-called interarticular bridge made of 8–10 mm thick soluble synthetic material which is provided by reinforced fiberglass embedded in a covering of synthetic resin. Without this bridge the ready-made shoe would become so deformed that the cosmetic demands would not be satisfied. In the case of male patients, as already pointed out above, the heel may be drawn down und forward, as shown in Figure 5. By this means, if necessary, more favorable proportions and dimensions can be attained and the wearing of ready-made shoes made possible. On the other hand, one must put up with the protruding heel, which would be quite disturbing if it could not be covered by a stocking. On this account, it can only be employed at best in the care of male patients.

Group c (14–30 cm leg length discrepancy)

Depending on the size of the leg length discrepancy and the specific clinical picture, and considering the sex of the patient and his/her cosmetic demands, several possibilities of design are available.

In male patients with leg length discrepancies of approx. 17 cm and up, the forefoot, placed in the most extreme equinus position, can be supported by a platform, as shown in Figure 6. There will be no further difficulty in retaining the dimensions of the artificial foot below so that ready-made shoes may be worn. Limb discrepancies of 10–16 cm in male patients may be treated similarly. The forefoot and toes can, of course, no longer be placed on a free-standing platform, which would have functional advantages, but must be so placed that the prosthesis or the inner shoe follows the essential configuration that will enable the patient to wear a ready-made shoe. This is illustrated clearly in Figure 12a. In these fabrications, any existing platform (see Fig. 6) or protruding heel (Fig. 12a) can be covered by a long stocking of sufficient width.

In women with leg discrepancies of this length, the cosmetic factors are of greater importance and the construction shown in Figure 6 cannot be employed. Operative measures should not be undertaken. The protruding heel can be padded to produce a better appearance. If this results in an unsightly discrepancy in calf circumference, then the heel can be completely covered, as shown in

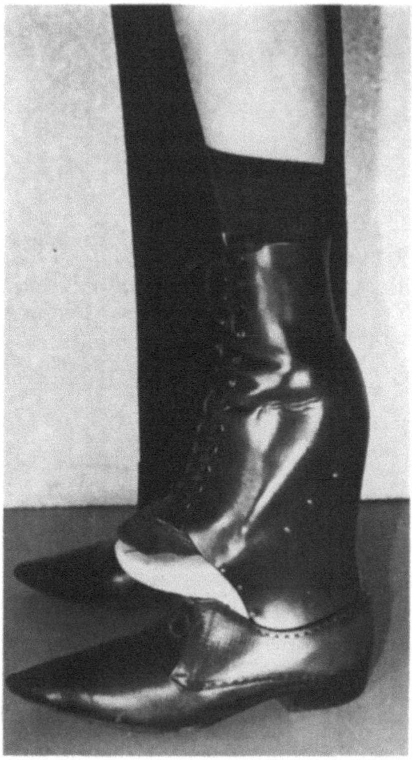

Fig. 6. "Elevator shoe" with the foot in marked equinus position and the forefoot propped up by a platform, in a discrepancy of 17 cm. Below, a prosthetic foot with a ready-made shoe. Cosmetically unsatisfactory. Suitable only for male patients

Figure 7. Fundamentally, the result is much more favorable if the foot can be placed in an extreme equinus position, which is in most cases possible in marked leg length discrepancies. Here the construction shown in Figure 3 can be employed – a method which leads to a completely satisfactory cosmetic result, which we shall discuss in detail below.

It should be added that obviously, when necessary, supplementary measures can be applied. These include supports on one or both sides of the ankle, braces, supporting flaps, tibial splints, peroneus spring devices or cosmetic repair of calf discrepancies.

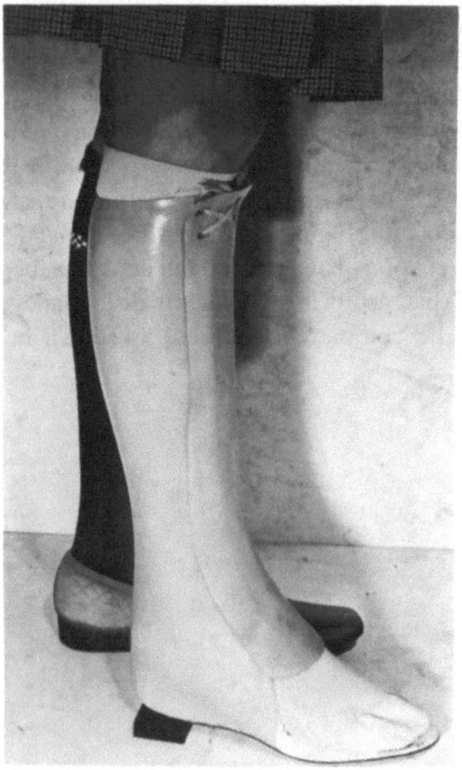

Fig. 7. Correction of shortened leg together with correction of a difference in the circumference of the calf. Cosmetic covering of the protruding heel

3. Principles of Measurement

Before taking measurements one must develop a clear plan for the construction of the prosthesis, and a working model must be executed. With regard to the physiologic and cosmetic aspects the primary consideration is to determine the optimal functional stabilization of the joints (Fig. 8). The following data and measures must be taken: the footprint, a foot and leg profile in the sagittal and vertical planes, a working diagram, and a plaster model.

With increase of the equinus position the ball of the big toe approaches the long axis of the lower leg. As a specific example, when the heel is raised 11 cm, and in a foot with a length of 27 cm, the ball of the foot approaches the long axis of the leg by 8 cm. This requires special consideration.

One must clearly understand that the equinus position leads to a substantial change in the statics and dynamics of walking. The size of the load is displaced forward from the heel to the detriment of the forefoot, while at the same time the overall supporting surface is decreased. Equinus also reduces the mechanically effective length of the forefoot. These factors must be compensated for functionally by the inner shoe. The equinus position is necessary if in equalizing leg lengths the cosmetic problem is to be worked out satisfactorily through use of a ready-made shoe. Both depend decisively on the forefoot positioning in the reparing of the plaster model.

With inner shoes for medium leg discrepancies of 6–10 cm, positioning must be correct within a matter of millimeters. In these cases the ball of the foot lies where normally, in a ready-made shoe, the shank is situated. In addition, construction of the inner shoe under the metatarsophalangeal joints calls for a thickness of 12–15 mm for the articular bridge and padding. Therefore, first of all a rough working sketch of the most favorable positioning of the foot is needed before undertaking the plaster model. Failure to do this will lead to errors of which two points should be emphasized.

1. Should the inner shoe under the ball of the foot be higher than necessary, the inevitable result is a foot that is too solid, clumsy, and cosmetically unsatisfactory. Moreover, the wearing of a ready-made shoe will be impossible.

2. The result is even worse if the forefoot is placed too low. In this case, there will be no room between the forefoot (weight-bearing surface of the ball) and the shoe for the inner shoe. To make an inner shoe from such a model would be a mistake, and were such an inner shoe to be placed in the shoe its position would not conform to the load axis of the upright leg. Such an inner shoe could not be worn.

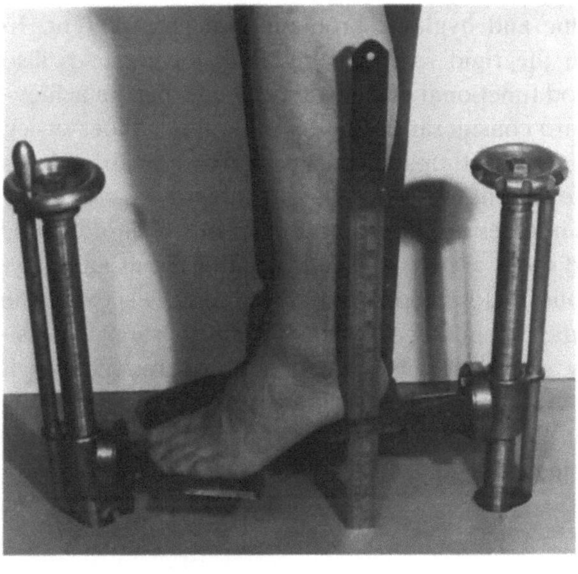

Fig. 8. Preparing to measure and make the plaster model. Determination of the optimal attitude of the joint

4. Possibilities of Improvement of Manufacturing Techniques with the Use of New Materials

As in the field of orthopaedics itself, new materials have opened new directions and possibilities in the manufacture of orthopaedic shoes. The rigid foam casting resin technique has proved to be particularly important. Inner shoes prepared by this technique are on the average 25% lighter than those made with the usual materials – not only lighter, but also more inherently stable and resistant to wear and tear. Moreover, the technique permits a thin-walled construction and thus a more form-fitting appliance, and – a decisive advantage – ready-made shoes may be worn. Open construction and perforations allow for ventilation. The fact that inner shoes made by the rigid foam casting resin technique may be easily cleaned is a real contribution to better hygiene. That inner shoes up to now have only been used to a limited extent is, in our own opinion, due predominantly to the fact that the rigid foam casting resin technique has not been made sufficiently known. The advantages of the rigid foam casting technique are evident when compared with the usual materials such as cork, leather, wood, rubber, felt, metal, and stiffening agents whose drawbacks include their weight, difficulties of maintaining combinations of material, lack of resistance to breaking and their relatively early deformation and inclination to cause sweating. Furthermore, with such materials one must put up with a very thick supporting base in order to offset the strong deforming forces. The result is an inner shoe that is heavy, clumsy, and functionally as well as esthetically unsatisfactory. The feet are altogether too "packed in," which, especially in warm weather, leads to heavy perspiration; simply on hygienic grounds such shoes become intolerable.

The improvements exhibited by the current techniques of inner shoe manufacture have contributed substantially to clarifying the indications in which they are preferable to conventional orthopaedic shoes. To be sure, the inner shoe has not simplified the technical problems with regard to manufacture; it has, however, answered the cosmetic and hygienic problem to a great extent. In principle, inner shoe care with the rigid foam casting resin technique is also practicable in children; very good functional and cosmetic results can be achieved. Of course, one must take into consideration the fact that inner shoes or leg lengthening prostheses are long-lived orthopaedic aids which on a financial basis have limited applicability for the patient whose foot is still growing.

The decision as to when inner shoes are appropriate and in which individual cases orthopaedically measured shoes are to be used instead of the usual ready-made shoe should be worked out in close cooperation between the specialist in orthopaedics and the orthopaedic shoemaker. Obviously, first the surgical possibilities have to be completely dealt with. But then, after operation, if it is obvious that orthopaedic shoe measures will still be necessary, it is desirable at the beginning of treatment that a combined plan of treatment be worked out in order to achieve the best possible result.

5. Special Inner Shoe Techniques in Limb Discrepancies of Approx. 6–13 cm

In all inner shoe treatment, leather always lies next to the skin; no other material has proved to be as compatible with skin. Therefore, a full leather cover has first to be applied to the plaster model and the pressure-sensitive areas provided with a 2–6 mm thick padding, e.g., beneath the metatarsal heads. Then the actual preparation can be carried out, with polyurethane or PVC rigid foam with a density of 0.08–0.18. By sanding, the preparation will be shaped so that it will fit loosely in the shoe. The face of the sole receives a thermically applied superimposed layer (stabilizer) of ortholen, 8–10 mm thick, which tapers down to the point of the inner shoe. With this a slight springiness is achieved and the ready-made shoe will hold its shape better in the area of the forefoot. The whole preparation, up to and including the top of the heel-plate, receives a coating of fiberglass-reinforced synthetic resin (casting resin). This coating is vitally important. It binds all the building materials together into a durable and wear-resistant article. Next comes a toe replacement of varying elasticity. At this point the inner shoe is tested. The trial must furnish clear information about the general fit and function of the inner shoe. Corrections are to be undertaken immediately and these checked by extensive walking tests, including walking on an uneven surface. Finally, the inner shoe is finished with a soft leather covering with a lace-up front. For several years, we have also been testing textile uppers, because they are lighter and airier than leather (Fig. 10). The inner shoe is now completed.

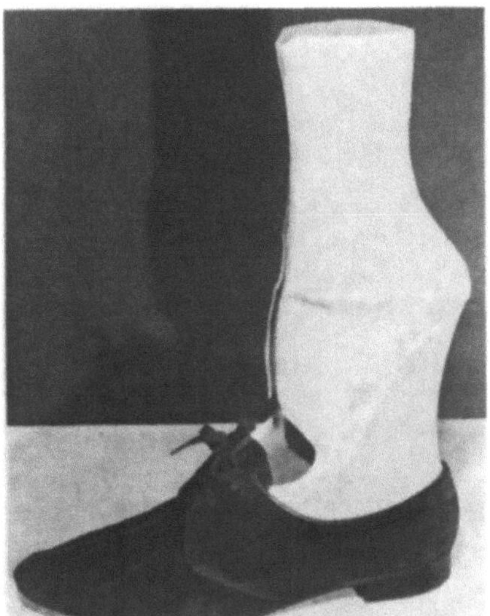

Fig. 9 A rough work-up of an inner shoe in a discrepancy of 10 cm, placed in a ready-made shoe

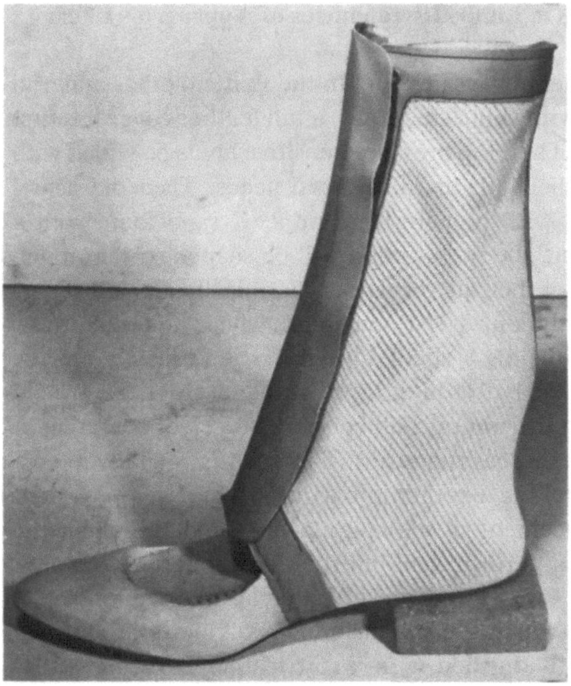

Fig. 10. Completed inner shoe with textile upper; lighter and better ventilated than leather

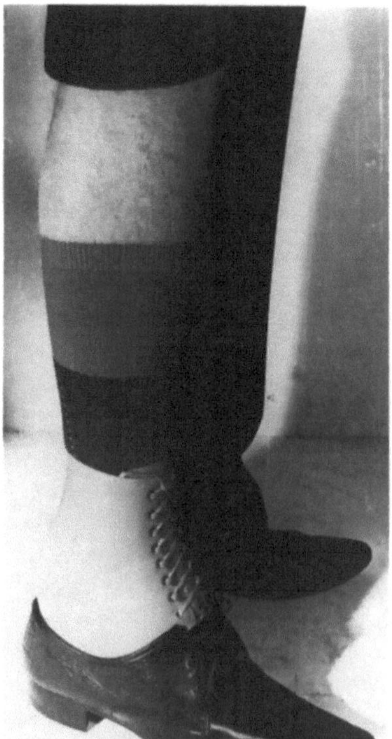

Fig. 11. Inner shoe in rigid foam casting resin technique in a discrepancy of 6.5 cm

II. Case Histories

To demonstrate the efficiency and advantages of the methods described above, the following case histories in which inner shoe prostheses have been used in our department are presented.

1. This was a right-sided leg shortening of 6.5 cm due to a childhood accident with damage to the proximal epiphyseal cartilage of the tibia. The right foot was easily brought into the equinus position; there was no significant malpositioning of the foot. A hard rubber casting resin inner shoe was fashioned, over which, as shown in Figure 11, a ready-made shoe of the patient's choice could be worn. Appropriately, a stocking should first be put on and the inner shoe worn over it. For cosmetic reasons, a second stocking can then be worn over the inner shoe. The weight of this inner shoe is 350 g. With normal clothing the foot is inconspicuous and cosmetically unobjectionable. The patient's gait is free and unhindered.

2. Here, the primary disease was a left-sided tuberculous coxitis during childhood. The left hip joint is firmly fused in a good functional position. In the course of growth there

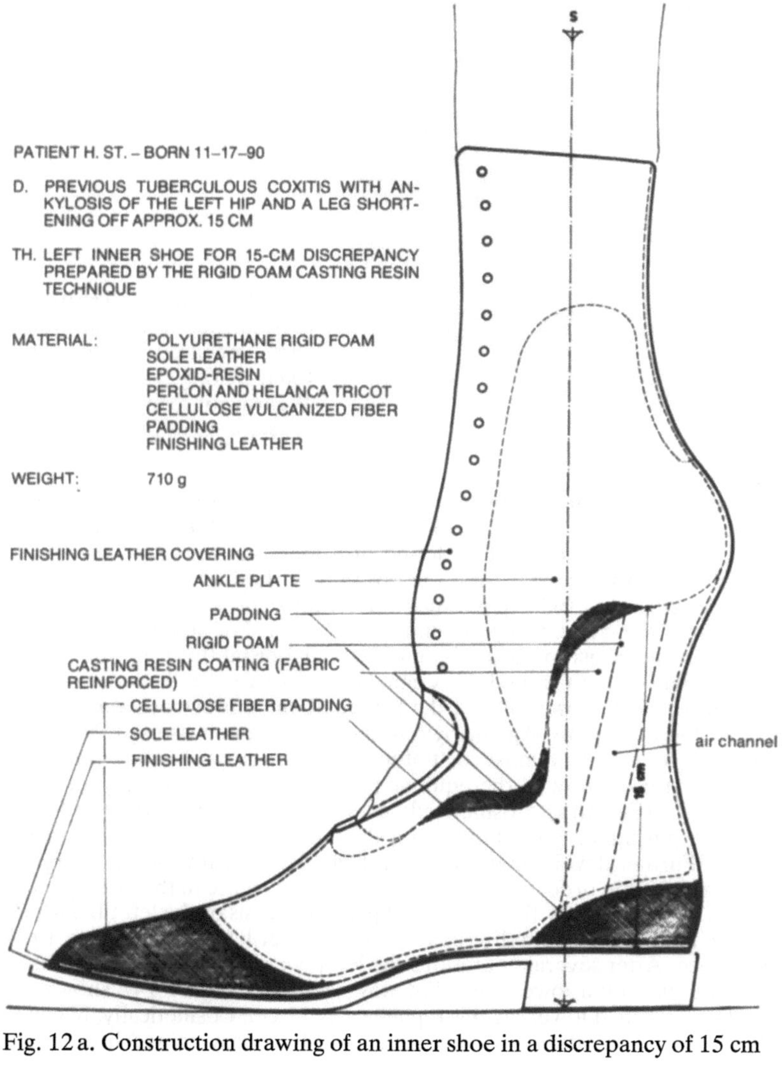

Fig. 12 a. Construction drawing of an inner shoe in a discrepancy of 15 cm

was an increasing discrepancy in the length of the left leg with considerable atrophy of the musculature. The earlier long-term immobilization of the leg, carried out on account of the tuberculous hip joint infection, has led secondarily to arthrotic changes of the left knee joint. In addition, the left foot was no longer freely movable but could, however, be brought into a sufficient equinus position. The total length discrepancy was 15 cm. Figure 12a is a construction drawing of an inner shoe to which the reader is referred for the technical details. Especially important in this case was the direction of the lines of the back of the foot so that the inner shoe would have the desired cosmetic profile. As illustrated in Figure 12b and c, ready-made shoes could be worn without difficulty; all together, a fully satisfactory cosmetic result was achieved. Also functionally the situation was good considering the ankylosis of the left hip joint. The weight of this rigid foam casting resin inner shoe was 710 g.

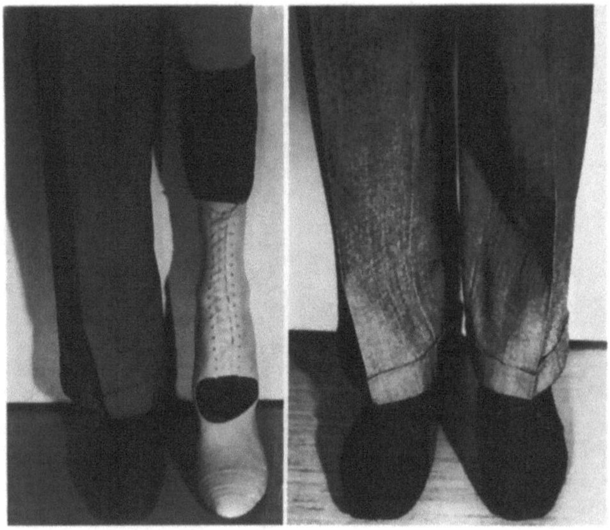

b c

Fig. 12b and c. Treatment carried out with the inner shoe prepared by the rigid foam casting resin technique. Wearing of ready-made shoes presents no difficulty

3. As already mentioned, it is thoroughly possible to fit children with inner shoes or leg lengthening prostheses. This girl, born in 1967, had right-sided fibula aplasia with a shortened tibia and aplasia of the entire fourth and fifth toes. As a result of the fibula aplasia a severe pes valgus was present. First the position of the foot was improved by appropriate tendon lengthening, following which an orthopaedic shoe procedure was carried out. At the time, the discrepancy amounted to 7.5 cm. For stabilization of the right lower leg, which at the transition from the middle to the distal third showed a mild anterior bowing with sclerosing of the medullary canal in this area – findings also seen in congenital pseudarthrosis of the lower leg –, the leg lengthening prosthesis was carried out up to the level of the knee joint. Again, rigid foam casting resin was used. We were successful in inserting the foot in almost a "tiptoe" position by cushioning the body weight under the heel with the foot in the equinus position. An appropriate prosthetic foot completed treatment (Fig. 13a). Cosmetically as well as functionally the result was very satisfactory. After putting on a stocking and a shoe, practically no pathologic signs are visible (Fig. 13b). Further development will reveal whether and at what time surgical intervention will be called for in order to correct the expected increase in the discrepancy.

4. This patient was born in 1940 with a congenital pseudarthrosis of the left tibia which with growth led to an increasing length discrepancy in the lower leg. From 1943 to 1945 he wore a long leg brace. After several operations the left lower leg was largely stabilized so that from that time on only a lower leg splint was necessary. Figure 14a shows the situation in 1966. The left-sided lower leg discrepancy was 12 cm. Cosmetically, hygienically, and functionally, the situation was unsatisfactory. It is easy to see how, using

materials like leather, wood, and cork, very strong metal splints must be fitted to obtain adequate stability. Also, one sees, primarily in the foot, the difficulty in getting a lasting union of the different materials. Preservation of shape and the problem of sweating are not solved. Figure 14 b shows the situation after care with an inner shoe made by the rigid foam casting resin technique. Preservation of shape is guaranteed, the leg lengthening prosthesis can be kept clean and hygienically faultless. The danger of damage through sweating does not exist. Cosmetically as well as functionally, the result is thoroughly satisfactory. Obviously, ready-made shoes can be worn. In contrast to the old splint apparatus, which weighed 1600 g, the new inner shoe weighs only 1050 g. Functionally, this saving of 550 g is without doubt valuable.

5. This girl was born in 1959 with a spina bifida in the sacral area and a meningocele, which was removed surgically during the first year of life. Histology revealed in addition a mixed tumor showing both neurofibromatous and lipomatous elements. There existed a

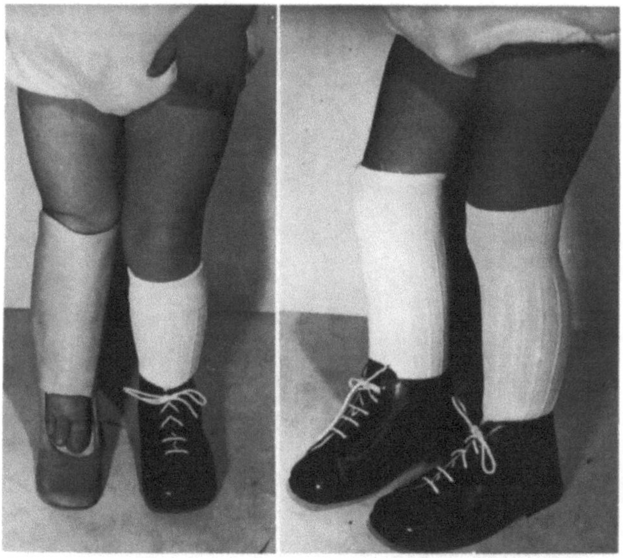

a b

Fig. 13a and b. Aplasia of fibula with aplasia of the 4th and 5th toes. Leg shortening of 7.5 cm. Leg lengthening prosthesis in rigid foam casting resin technique

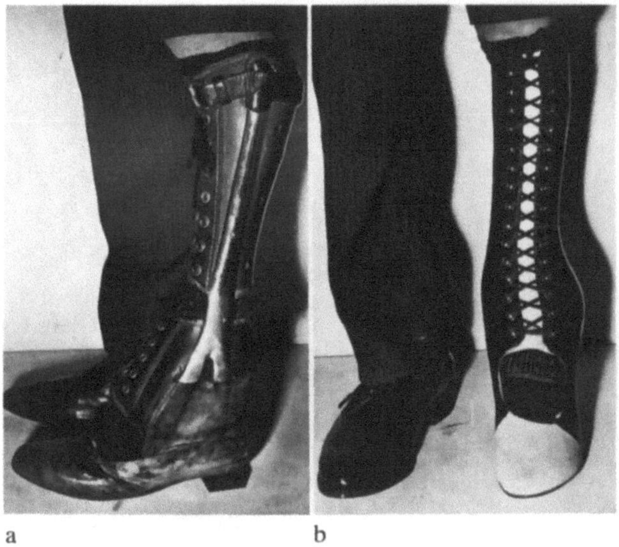

a b

Fig. 14a and b. Left tibial pseudarthrosis with lower leg discrepancy of 12 cm. Previously treated by cork-leather technique with metal splints; re-treated with inner shoe by rigid foam casting resin technique partial paralysis of the left leg combined with considerable trophic disturbances, left-sided leg shortening, and a severe talipes deformity of the left foot (Fig. 15a). Owing to this situation, she was fitted with a lower leg splint and an orthopaedic boot to equalize the leg length discrepancy, (Fig. 15b), measures which were of limited value both functionally and cosmetically. In treatment, first of all the malposition of the left foot was corrected surgically and at the same time the foot was set in a slight equinus position. Next, an inner shoe was prepared according to the rigid foam casting resin technique together with an ankle support. Because of the patient's age we could not consider an arthrodesis of the ankle joint (Fig. 15c). However, now the cosmetic result is substantially better than before (Fig. 15d). Whereas the old lower leg splint with orthopaedic boot weighed 925 g, the weight of the inner shoe and shoe is 515 g. The girl herself was very happy with the result. With further operative measures in the near future, the situation will be even more favorable.

a b

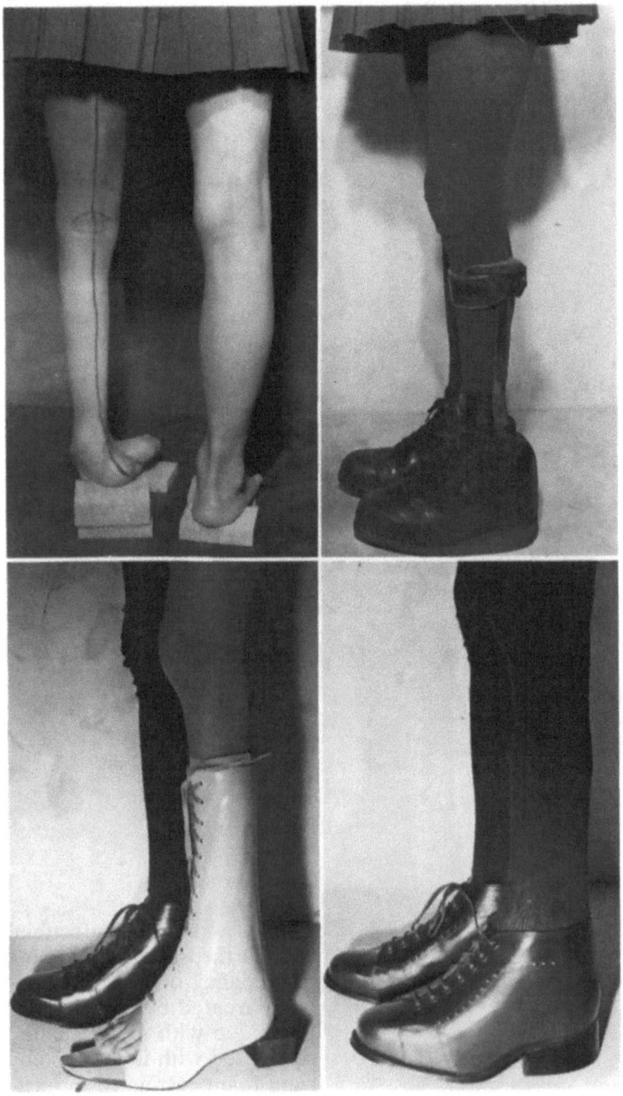

c d

Fig. 15a–d. Partial left leg paralysis with talipes deformity and leg shortening. Previously fitted with lower leg splint and orthopaedic boots; after foot surgery patient was fitted with inner shoe by rigid foam casting resin technique

6. Born in 1943, this patient contracted poliomyelitis in 1945. He was left with paresis of the left quadriceps muscle, an extensive paresis of the musculature of the left lower leg with equinovarus of the left foot, and a leg shortening of 6 cm (Fig. 16 a). As a result, he was treated with a short leg splint and apparatus to compensate for the discrepancy. He was able to wear ready-made shoes. However, the apparatus was heavy and hygienically unsatisfactory (Fig. 16 b). Therefore, an inner shoe was prepared according to the rigid foam casting resin technique and, because of the extensive pareses, included a high shaft. An operation which might well have improved the situation was refused by the patient. But, as Figures 16 c and d show, a cosmetically satisfactory picture was achieved by conservative measures. The weight of the apparatus was reduced from 1460 g to 890 g and the hygienic situation considerably improved. Also functionally the result was considered very good.

7. In this case it is a matter of the sequelae of a left-sided tuberculous coxitis of childhood. The left hip joint is in a slightly flexed position and solidly ankylosed. Secondary arthrotic changes in the area of the left knee joint resulted from a lengthy immobilization in a plaster cast so that today full extension is no longer possible. The left foot, however, has only minor limitation of movement. The left leg discrepancy is 20.5 cm. The patient was first fitted with a splint apparatus with a corresponding correction of the

a b

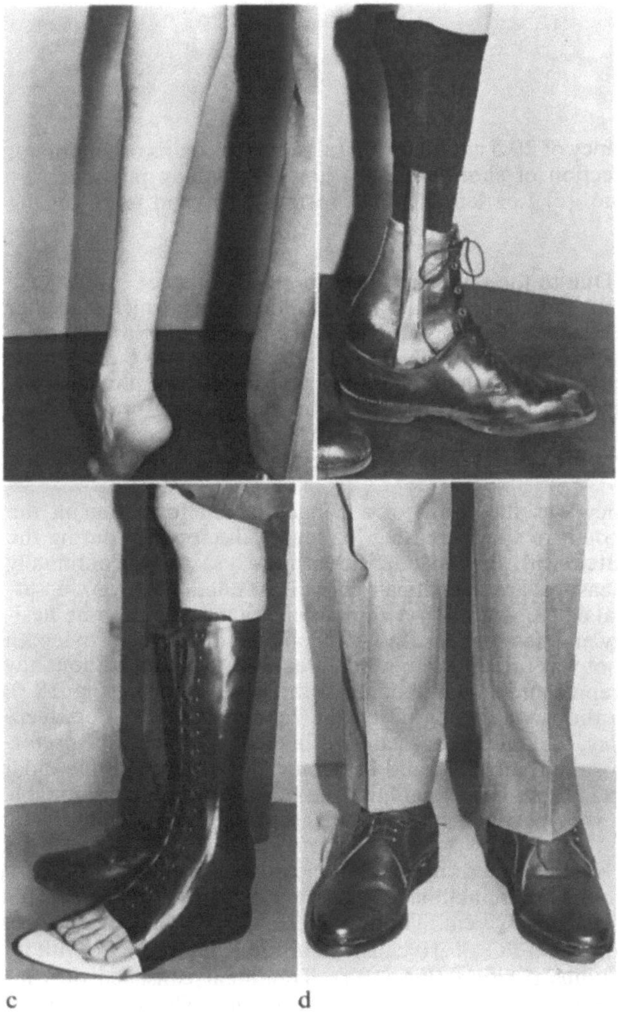

c d

Fig. 16 a–d. Extensive paralysis of the left leg with a shortening of 6 cm and faulty foot position following poliomyelitis. Previously cared for with a lower leg splint apparatus, now with an inner shoe made by the rigid foam casting resin technique

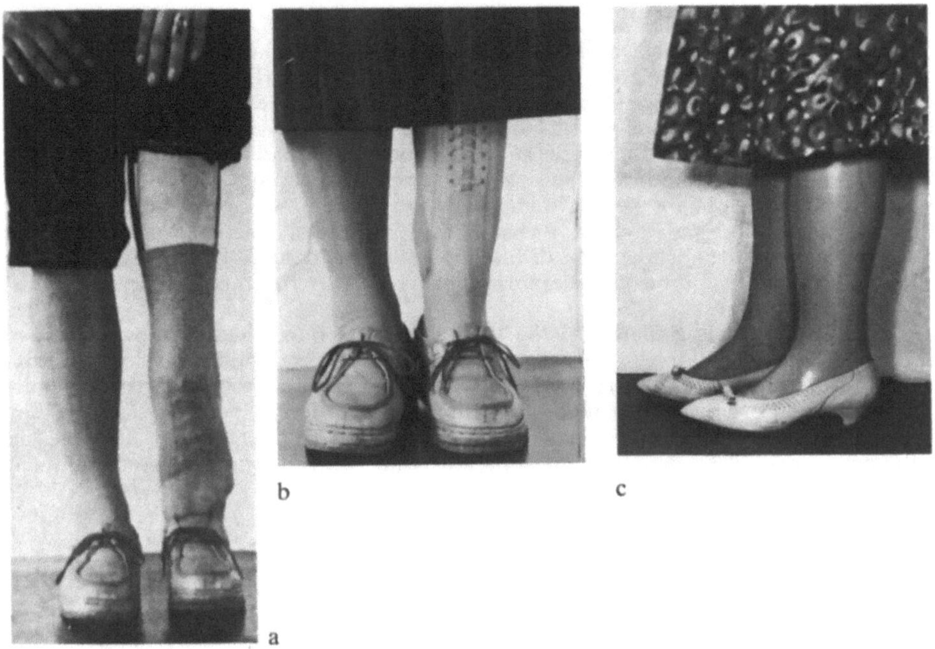

Fig. 17 a–c. Left-sided discrepancy of 20.5 cm following tuberculous coxitis of childhood. (a) Splint apparatus with correction of shortening. (b) Leg lengthening prosthesis by leather-rubber-Bofors technique. (c) Leg lengthening prosthesis by rigid foam casting resin technique

length discrepancy (Fig. 17a). Due to the unfavorable cosmetic appearance caused by a deficiency in covering the foot, the patient had to always wear long pants, which made her very unhappy. Hence, in 1956 a leg lengthening prosthesis was prepared by the leather-rubber-Bofors technique (Fig. 17b). In comparison to the previous state, the cosmetic situation was clearly improved; on the other hand the still visible lacing was quite disturbing. Only by the rigid foam casting resin technique can a leg lengthening prosthesis be prepared that not only functionally but above all also cosmetically can be labelled good (Fig. 17c). It is always gratifying to observe the positive psychological effect on the patient.

8. Here a left leg discrepancy was the result of a congenital malformation in the proximal femoral area. On account of the increasing leg length discrepancy during the early years the patient was fitted with orthopaedic boots that had to be continually readjusted. These customary measures are cosmetically as well as functionally very unsatisfactory. Frequently, the actual discrepancy is not completely balanced since one hesitates to make increasingly bulky and heavy shoes. In later years the discrepancy in length amounted to 18 cm. The left foot was brought into marked equinus position without any difficulty so that it practically represented a lengthening of the axis of the leg (Fig. 18a). In 1960 a leg lengthening prosthesis was prepared by the rubber-leather-Bofors technique (Fig. 18b). Although today, the rigid foam casting resin technique would be preferred, nevertheless quite good cosmetic success could be achieved at times with the older technique. The patient was able to fulfil her long-cherished desire to wear fashionable pumps. Figure 18c shows that even vogues such as spike heels present no difficulties with such prostheses.

9. This patient, born in 1939, contracted in early infancy osteomyelitis of the right lower leg with severe damage to the proximal tibial epiphyseal cartilage. With growth, the discrepancy increased, finally reaching 22 cm. The mobility of the left knee joint was limited to 120° of flexion with an FFC of 10°. The left foot was brought without difficulty into the maximal equinus position (Fig. 19a). Treatment consisted of a leg lengthening prosthesis made by the rigid foam casting resin technique. The outer shape of

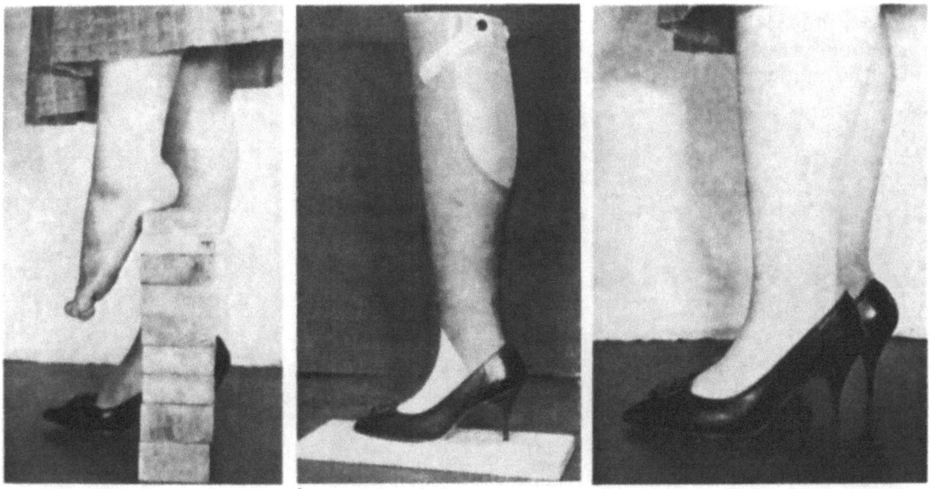

a b c

Fig. 18a–c. Left-sided discrepancy of 18 cm in partial aplasia of the femur. Leg lengthening prosthesis by leather-rubber-Bofors technique

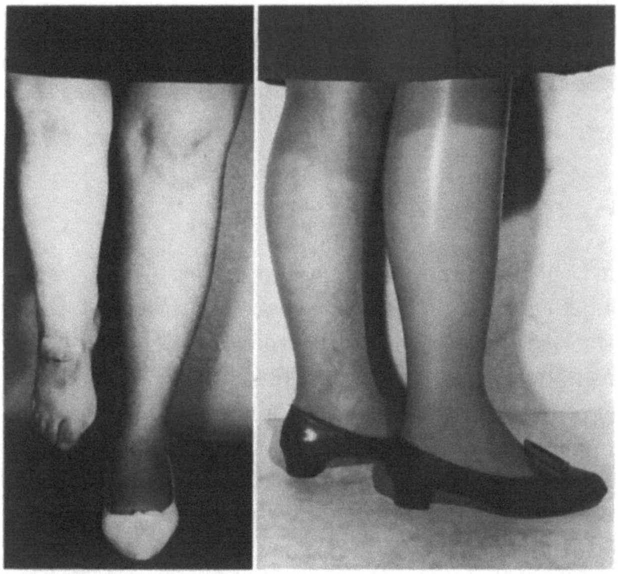

a b

Fig. 19a and b. Infantile osteomyelitis of the right tibia with a lower leg shortening of 22 cm. Treated with a leg lengthening prosthesis by the rigid foam casting resin technique

this prosthesis matches the left leg so that all together, the cosmetic result is very satisfactory (Fig. 19b).

10. This patient has a malformation in the right leg with a length discrepancy that reached 27 cm by the end of growth. An orthopaedic shoe was prepared with a length compensation of 17 cm (Fig. 20a). In spite of this very clumsy and cosmetically unacceptable shoe the discrepancy in length was not equalized, the remaining deficit being 10 cm. Accordingly, in standing, the left knee joint had to be bent in an attempt to correct for the inadequacy of the treatment. Moreover, the patient had a marked pelvic tilt to the right with a corresponding strain on the spinal column. Even though the therapeutic goal was in no way achieved, evidently no one had dared to build a higher shoe, which would surely have been rejected by the patient because of its weight and ugliness. Here also a leg lengthening prosthesis was prepared with the rigid foam casting resin technique with

full correction of the 27-cm discrepancy. The patient became from one minute to the next 10 cm taller. The functional result was very favorable. General statics have been restored and the cosmetic result is unobjectionable (Fig. 20b).

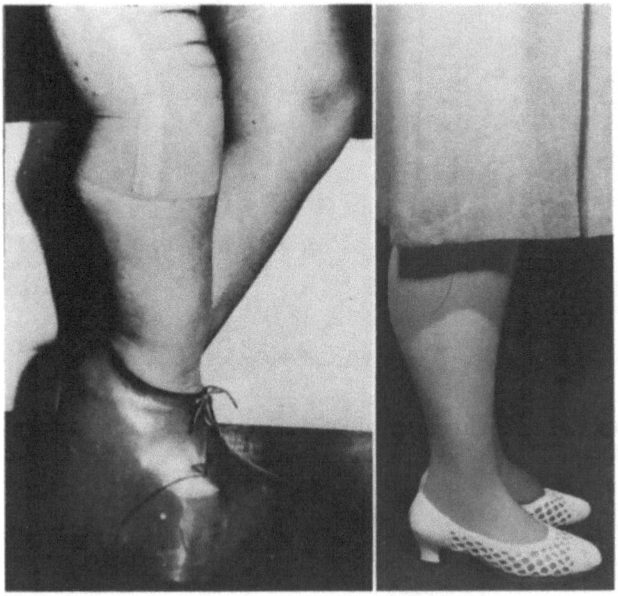

a b

Fig. 20a and b. Congenital malformation of the right leg with shortening of 27 cm. Inadequate care with orthopaedic boots to correct discrepancy. Newly treated with a leg lengthening prosthesis by the rigid foam casting resin technique

III. Concluding Remarks

It may be definitely said that with the orthopaedic shoe methods and the well-known materials and techniques available today, especially the rigid foam casting resin technique, conservative treatment of differences in leg length can produce functionally and cosmetically satisfactory results. These orthopaedic shoe techniques consequently represent an important supplement to the surgical correction of these discrepancies. As matters stand, by virtue of the primary disease, not all differences in leg length are fully amenable to surgery, and there will always be a certain percentage of patients who shy away from surgery and prefer conservative treatment. It must, however, be remembered that successful inner shoe care represents a craftsman's art and is regarded today as a particularly valuable qualification of an orthopaedic shoemaker. Obviously, the new materials need further observation and development, while the manufacturing techniques require constant refinement. The orthopaedic shoe techniques that are now available for correction of leg length discrepancies are still not widely appreciated or extensively used. However, the results achieved in this field and the experience acquired to date clearly demonstrate that the inner shoe represents a genuine advantage over previous methods of care. Therefore, it would appear to be desirable that education and training in these special techniques be extended. In spite of progress in operative treatment there will in the future be no small demand for properly trained orthopaedic shoemakers.

Summary

Essentially, there are three different methods available today for correction of leg length discrepancies with the use of orthopaedic shoe techniques. Firstly, in discrepancies of up to approx. 2.5 cm, ready-made shoes can be converted by raising the heel or the heel and the sole, and, if necessary, also by fitting in a 6–10 mm thick cork support in the shoe.

Secondly, there is the usual orthopaedic footwear in which the correction is built into and becomes a part of the orthopaedic shoe. Finally, there is the possibility of the inner shoe, or, in extreme length differences, the so-called leg lengthening prosthesis. In these cases, ready-made shoes can usually be worn. Since the conversion of ready-made shoes and orthopaedic footwear with built-in correction are well known, inner shoe methods of treatment and leg lengthening prostheses are discussed in detail, specifically with regard to indications and technical problems with particular consideration given to the use of new materials. Illustrative case histories also are presented.

References

Meyer, E.: Orthopädieschuhm.-Handwerk **6,** 186–192 (1966)
Meyer, E.: Orthopädieschuhmachermeister **3,** 57–61 (1967)
Meyer, E.: Orthopädieschuhmachermeister **10,** 334–337 (1968)
Petersen, D.: Münch. med. Wschr. **111,** 791–798 (1969)

English translation from the German edition *Der Orthopäde,* Vol. 1, pp. 21–34 (1972),

Subtrochanteric Shortening and Lengthening Osteotomy

P. Heidensohn, D. Hohmann, and M. Weigert*

Codevilla (1905) was the first to report femoral lengthening osteotomy. Because of a growing awareness of the potential complications coupled with the requisite precautions, particularly slow distraction rates, and with better definition of the indications, this procedure has become significantly less risky. However, the gain in length that can be attained without danger with this procedure is at most 4–5 cm.

Ample lengthening of the long bones of 10–15 cm and more may be achieved with Anderson's continuous distraction technique and with the recent technical improvements introduced by Wagner. As a rule, these methods require an additional plate osteosynthesis and cancellous bone grafting, but because they preserve height and bodily proportions, they are, in extreme leg length discrepancies, the treatments of choice (Wagner).

Here we shall not report on lengthenings of such spectacular scale, but rather describe a simple, low-risk modification of femoral length equalization that employs a combination of well-known methods. Primarily, this technique comes under consideration when a correction of from 5 to about 10 cm is called for. The principle of the procedure consists of shifting the combined shortening and lengthening osteotomies of Lezius and Lange from the middle of the shaft to the immediate subtrochanteric area. There are several reasons for this:

1. Fixation of the shortened femur with an intramedullary nail sometimes does not turn out to provide reliable stability, because a substantial quantity of medullary canal is lost through resection of the bone segment and there are limits to the amount of intramedullary reaming (Goff; Taillard and Morscher; Lange; Müller; Viernstein and Weigert).

2. In the shortened and usually hypoplastic femur there exists to begin with a distinct difference in caliber between the transplant from the longer side and the shortened femur. Therefore, here also, reaming does not always lead to an

* Orthopädische Klinik mit Poliklinik der Universität Erlangen–Nuremberg, Federal Republic of Germany (Director: Prof. Dr. med. D. Hohmann), und Orthopädische Klinik mit Poliklinik der Freien Universität Berlin im Oskar-Helene-Heim (Director: Prof. Dr. med. G. Friedebold)

intramedullary osteosynthesis that is rotationally stable. An additional immobilization in a spica cast cannot always be avoided. This is particularly disadvantageous because of the importance of early mobilization of the knee, already the site of soft tissue abnormalities due to the lengthening or shortening procedure.

3. The cortical bone of a mid-shaft osteotomy consolidates very slowly. Likewise, healing of the translocated cortical bone segment into the cortex of the lengthened side is usually considerably delayed. Pseudarthroses are not uncommon.

As a rule, a shortening osteotomy in the partly cancellous subtrochanteric area is relatively quickly consolidated so that after 6 weeks the side has its full weight bearing capacity. In addition, the bone cylinder taken from the longer side is richer in cancellous bone and becomes revascularized much more quickly in the partly cancellous tissue into which it is inserted.

The distraction should be accomplished with a single supracondylar Steinmann pin; the danger of infection is then minimal. Double distraction instruments, such as Küntscher's distractors, which are used with large Kirschner wires, not infrequently lead to pin tract infections, particularly in the proximal end of the femur where the soft tissues are so abundant. The supracondylar pin, on the other hand, lies distant from the subtrochanteric site of operation.

Certain difficulties can arise in lengthenings of more than 4 cm due to axial deviation of the fragments resulting from asymmetric soft-tissue tension. These and also rotational deformities can be avoided by inserting a pertrochanteric or condylar plate, before the lengthening osteotomy and application of traction. A sliding plate screwed onto the distal fragment exactly in the axis of the femur maintains the relative position of the distal fragment. If the shortening osteotomy is carried out at the first operation, one can insert the removed bone cylinder into the musculature on the side to be lengthened. This cylinder is then transferred into the defect where distraction is complete. Whether this results in quicker healing is not proved. One disadvantage is that the degree of shortening is already fixed at the first operation so that if an infection should occur in the site being distracted or the distraction does not attain its projected length, an exact correction of the discrepancy cannot under those circumstances be realized. For this reason, we perform the shortening osteotomy only at the second operation and after attaining the desired distraction on the opposite side and thus implant the bone cylinder directly into the defect produced by lengthening.

Fixation after transfer of the subtrochanteric bone cylinder from the shortened to the elongated side follows by means of an angle plate or condylar plate compression osteosynthesis. This allows early exercise and weight bearing since the healing time will be shortened. The restriction on lengthening to 4–5 cm obviates the danger of traction damage (sciatic nerve paralysis, muscle weakness, vascular damage) (Fig. 1).

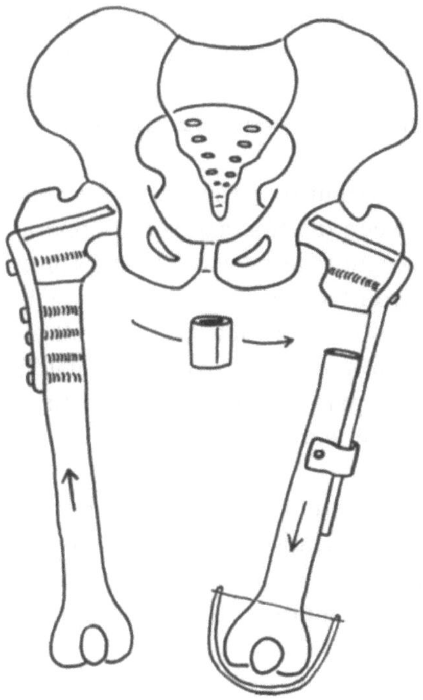

Fig. 1. Schematic diagram of the operative procedure. Subtrochanteric shortening osteotomy on the left, immobilized with a compression plate. Subtrochanteric lengthening osteotomy with insertion of the cylinder on the right. Supracondylar distraction

Technique of Operation

At the first operation the condylar or pertrochanteric plate is fixed to the neck of the elongated femur and a horizontal osteotomy is carried out in the distal third of the lesser trochanter. A guiding plate is attached to the distal fragment of the femur through which the shaft of the condylar plate can glide. The guiding plate is attached to the shaft with 2–4 short cortical screws. A Steinmann pin is inserted in the supracondylar region to which the distraction bow is attached. After closing the wound the patient is placed in bed, with the foot of the bed elevated. Increasing traction with weights of up 20 kg follows under X-ray control, initially every 2 or 3 days and then once a week. Daily examination of neural and vascular function is necessary. Upon attaining the desired distraction, a subtrochanteric shortening osteotomy is carried out on the other leg using an AO-angle compression plate in the subtrochanteric area. The bone cylinder is then transferred to the previously distracted site. Heavy-duty self-retaining distracting forceps have proved useful in this phase of the operation. Insertion of the cylinder is followed by compression osteosynthesis and fixation with screws. Rotation is assured by the guiding plate which is only removed after fixation with the screws. Before a final fixation another check is made to see that the legs are of equal length.

A leg length discrepancy of 6–7 cm can also be a one-stage operation. First, the lengthening osteotomy is carried out and the limb distracted some 2–3 cm. Next, the shortening osteotomy is carried out with removal of the bone implant, and last the final lengthening and insertion of the bone cylinder is carried out.

To date, this procedure has been employed by us in six patients between the ages of 18 and 30 years. The time elapsed between the first and second operation averaged 2–3 weeks; the time to partial weight bearing was 12 weeks after the first operation. Full weight bearing was permitted on an average 16 weeks after the first operation. The leg length correction was successful in all six patients operated on. Differences of between 6 and 10 cm were eliminated. Consolidation was in no case delayed. No nerve paralysis, blood flow disturbances, ankyloses, or other traction damages were observed.

We recommend that the osteosynthesis plates used in these free bone transplants not be removed before $1^1/_2$–2 years from operation. At another institution plates removed after about 1 year led, despite an X-ray appearance of complete consolidation, to a fracture at the distal margin of the transplanted fragment.

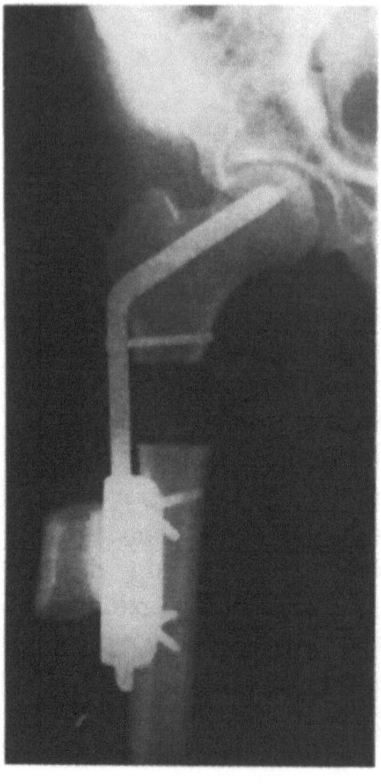

Fig. 2. Sliding plate. Distraction about 4 cm. The bone cylinder from the opposite side has been embedded in the vastus lateralis muscle

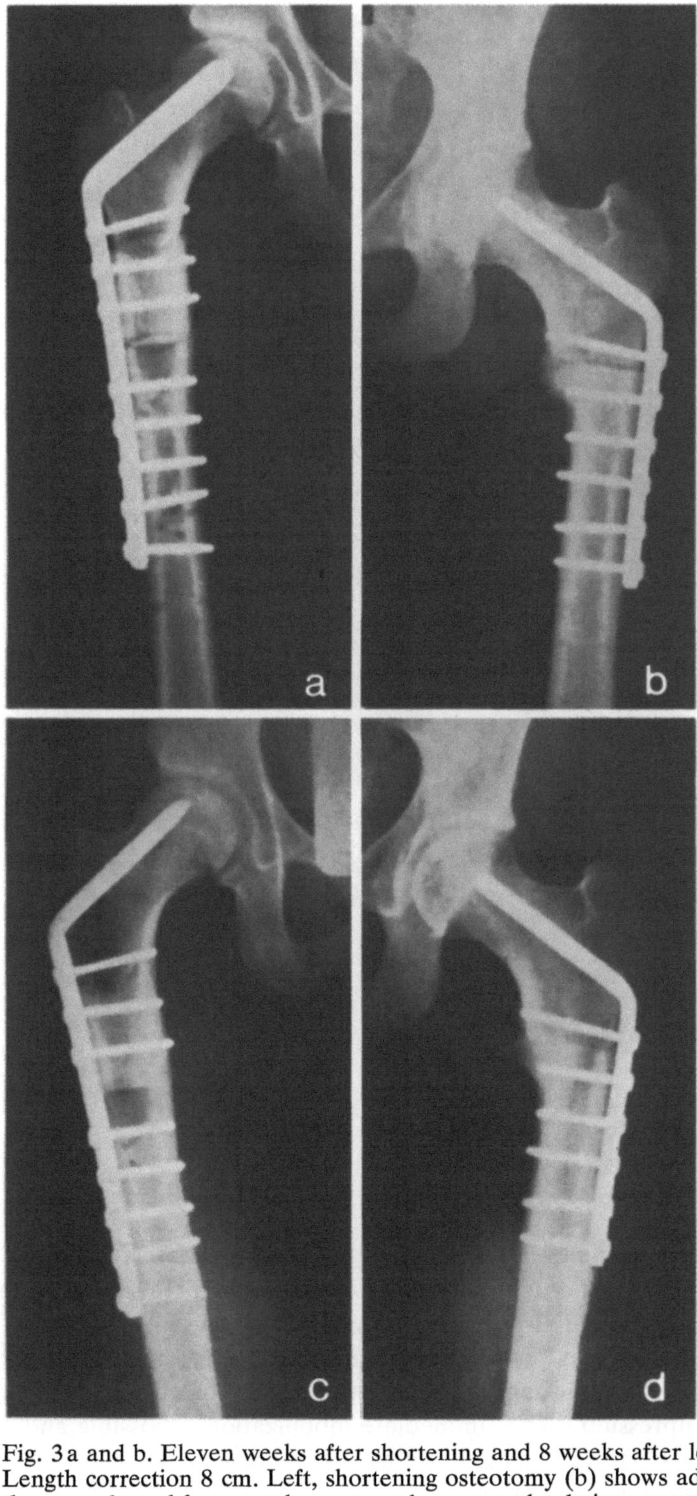

Fig. 3a and b. Eleven weeks after shortening and 8 weeks after lengthening osteotomy. Length correction 8 cm. Left, shortening osteotomy (b) shows advancing healing, while the transplanted fragment has not yet been completely incorporated. (c) and (d) Osteotomy 6 months after operation; both sides essentially consolidated

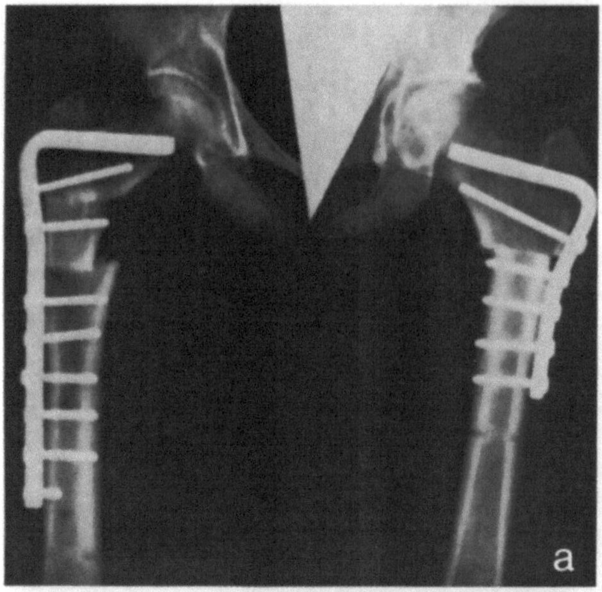

Fig. 4a. Osteotomy 6 weeks after the second operation. Length correction 7.5 cm

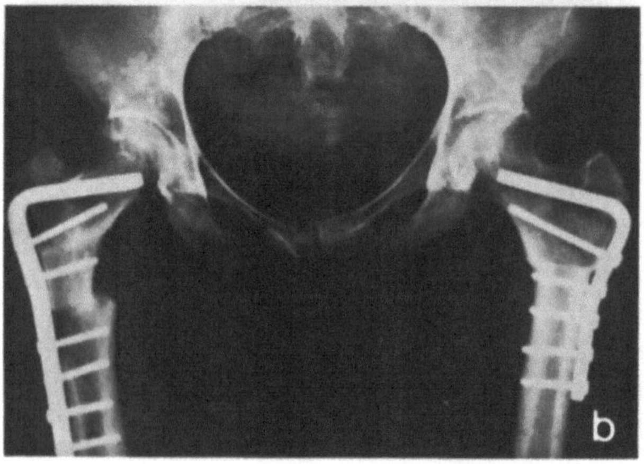

Fig. 4b. Osteotomies 4 months after the second operation. Both sides show bony union

Summary

In this procedure of shortening and lengthening osteotomy for correction of length discrepancies of the upper leg, the danger of infection in the subtrochanteric area of the upper leg is considerably reduced through use of the supracondylar distraction pin. During distraction the fragments are guided precisely through the sliding plate. By shifting the osteotomy to the subtrochanteric area and fixation with compression plates, immediate mobilization is possible and a plaster cast superfluous. Moreover, the exact axial alignment of both femora is guaranteed and a rapid consolidation of the osteotomies is enhanced. Due to the slow distraction and its limited extent, the danger of traction damage is minimal.

References

Anderson, W. V.: J. Bone Jt Surg. **34 B,** 150 (1952)
Codevilla, A.: Amer. J. orthop. Surg. **2,** 353 (1905)
Goff, Ch. W.: Surgical treatment of unequal extremities. Springfield, Ill.: Ch. C Thomas 1960
Lange, M.: Orthopädisch-chirurgische Operationslehre, 2. Aufl.: Erg.-Bd.: Neueste Operationsverfahren. München: Bergmann 1968
Lezius, A.: Chirurg **17/18,** 162 (1946/47)
Müller, M. E.: Die hüftnahen Femurosteotomien, 2. Aufl. Stuttgart: Thieme 1971
Taillard, W., Morscher, E.: Die Beinlängenunterschiede. Basel–New York: Karger 1965
Viernstein, K., Weigert, M.: Münch. med. Wschr. **109,** 666 (1967)
Wagner, H.: Chirurg **42,** 260 (1971)

English translation from the German edition *Der Orthopäde,* Vol. 1, pp. 46–49 (1972),

Surgical Lengthening or Shortening of Femur and Tibia. Technique and Indications

H. Wagner*

Any lower limb length discrepancy results in marked impairment of form and function of the locomotor system. It influences the patterns of gait and causes abnormal stresses and dysfunctions of the joints of the spine and lower limb. Leg length discrepancies of more than 4 cm represent a severe disturbance, while lesser differences are frequently better tolerated. Some patients can compensate a shortening of 2 to 3 cm with ease. Others respond with abnormal body posture, unphysiologic gait patterns and pain. The latter require corrective measures.

Some patients with leg length difference are affected psychologically by its aesthetic consequences, such as the asymmetry of their body proportions, the unequal position of their knee joints while walking or sitting and a noticeably short leg limb. It should be mentioned that a large number of these patients look at a lower limb discrepancy as a defect which seems to annoy them more than other comparable deformities. They are willing to make great sacrifices for their correction or concealment. The indication for correction must include aesthetic as well as physiological factors.

Lower limb discrepancies can be treated by conservative means; for example, by lifts put on regular shoes, by orthopaedic shoes with special adjustments, or by inlays, braces and orthotic devices. Conservative methods are limited in their use, even though they will have to be employed in particular circumstances. Two essential disadvantages cannot be overcome in the more significant leg length discrepancies.

1. The knee joints remain at different levels if the shortening is in the femur. Corrective aids can only be placed under the foot, not at the true site of shortening. This leaves functional and aesthetic problems unsolved.

2. Such aids used to correct the larger limb length discrepancies become increasingly bulky and clumsy. Finally, they become totally objectionable from the cosmetic appearance alone. Staining of these aids due to sweating, the

* Orthopädische Klinik des Wichernhauses Nuremberg/Altdorf (Head Physician: Prof. Dr. H. Wagner), Federal Republic of Germany

resultant odor combined with the limited possibility for cleaning adds to the discomfort of their wearers.

Female patients are particularly distressed by these aesthetic factors. Wearing modern dresses or a bathing suit causes embarassement which may lead to major psychological problems. Marked lower limb leg discrepancies can even influence the chance of finding a spouse. Leg length equalization by an aesthetically, hygienically unsatisfactory prosthesis hardly improves the chances.

Experience has taught us that many patients, particularly women, have strong adverse psychological reactions against even the most modern aids, sometimes more so than against the deformity itself. Frequently they decline to wear any of these orthopaedic paraphernalia.

In trying to camouflage the discrepancy, these patients tend to walk and stand with their affected foot in plantar flexion, and with a pelvic tilt, and by flexing the hip and knee joint of the opposite extremity. They can be quite successful in masking even significant discrepancies by these means, but do not realize the long-term effect such compensating measures have on the adjacent joints, and particularly the lumbar discs.

We have seen young women who declined any prosthetic help in spite of leg length discrepancies of 20 cm and who ambulated in an extremely unphysiological manner. We shall not try to analyse this abnormal physiological behavior. It is possible that prior errors in education or therapy are responsible for their reaction. All we intend to do is to stress the fact that the use of technical aids can produce psychological problems. From this it becomes evident that the indication for conservative lower limb discrepancy correction depends not only on the availability of othopaedic aids but, much more so, on the willingness of the patient to wear them.

These previously mentioned problems are not a phenomenon of our times but today's patients expect more as far as their rehabilitation is concerned. Even in times past the need has been felt for a surgical correction of leg length discrepancy either by lengthening of the affected leg or shortening of the unaffected side. Many such attempts have been carried out with varying degrees of success. However, only recently, and in particular since the development of effective osteosynthesis, has the problem of surgical lengthening of the shortened leg been so satisfactorily solved that most patients can be offered the possibility of complete or near complete surgical correction of their discrepancy.

Older surgical methods employing forced distraction, frequently resulting in soft tissue, vascular and nerve damage, or methods which required bed rest for many months, have become outmoded. Today we have very efficient techniques for correcting leg length discrepancies without any long-term immobilization. Their effectiveness has been proved on many patients.

The following operations can be recommended:

A. Surgery Involving the Longer Limb

1. Metaphyseal shortening osteotomies with osteosynthesis
   a) Femoral
   b) Tibial
2. Diaphyseal shortening osteotomies with intra- or extra-medullary osteosynthesis
   a) Femoral
   b) Tibial

B. Surgery Involving the Shorter Limb

1. One-stage metaphyseal femoral elongation osteotomies with osteosynthesis and cancellous bone grafting, if necessary with correction of axial deformities.
2. One-stage diaphyseal elongation osteotomies, with osteosynthesis and cancellous bone grafting.
   a) Femoral
   b) Tibial
3. Diaphyseal elongation osteotomies employing continuous distraction and if necessary cancellous bone grafting followed by osteosynthesis
   a) Femoral
   b) Tibial

Any one of these operations can be accomplished with today's techniques and they are of equal value. Each method has limited indications, advantages and disadvantages. Jointly they represent the spectrum of possible modern operative correction. Each patient who requires such an operation has to be evaluated individually, and all individual factors must be considered in selecting the proper operative method or appropriate combinations.

A. Operations on the Longer Lower Extremity

1 a) Metaphyseal Shortening Osteotomies of the Femur

This is the most effective method of all operations which try to correct limb length discrepancies by shortening the longer limb. Its most common site is the proximal femoral metaphysis, numerically followed by osteotomies at the distal femoral metaphysis.

Shortening osteotomies of the proximal femoral metaphysis: The fascia lata is split longitudinally from a lateral approach. This is followed by detaching the vastus lateralis muscle from the lateral border of the greater trochanter and the linea aspera. The femur is exposed subperiosteally. A hole is made in the lateral cortex of the greater trochanter for the seating device for a right-angle osteosynthesis plate which is then inserted into the trochanter-neck area.

In cases requiring shortening only the seating device is inserted at a right angle to the femoral shaft. Correction of axial deformities requires proper orientation of the seating device. Next, the distance to be shortened is outlined on the bone. Application of longitudinal markers for control of rotatory correction is necessary. Next, the bone is osteotomized distally. The necessary amount of bone is excised proximally by using a bone saw. A part of the medial cortex in continuity with the trochanter minor is left intact (Fig. 1A). This creates a right-angle surface which allows wide contact with the distal osteotomy site. Apposition of the fragments is then carried out and stabilization of the osteotomy site is obtained by employing the osteotomy plate. The advantages of this method as compared to more distal operations are that it is performed in an area of minor soft tissue mobility and therefore causes no impairment of joint function.

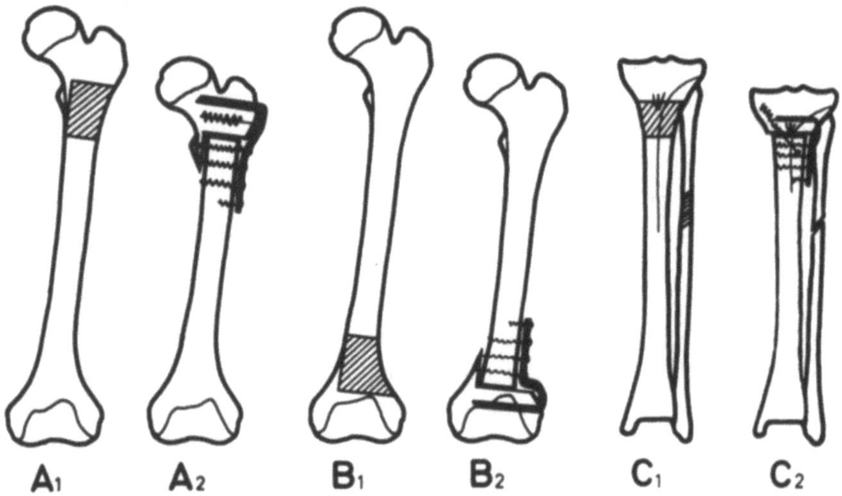

Fig. 1. Metaphyseal shortening osteotomy of femur and tibia (areas of resection are hatched). A_1 Amount and site of intertrochanteric shortening osteotomy. A_2 Coaptation of fragments with wide area of contact, compression osteosynthesis. B_1 Amount and site of supracondylar shortening osteotomy. B_2 Coaptation of fragments, compression osteosynthesis. C_1 Amount and site for metaphyseal tibio-fibular shortening osteotomy. C_2 Coaptation of fragments, compression osteosynthesis

Shortening osteotomy of the distal femoral metaphysis: Shortening osteotomies of the distal femoral metaphysis are carried our in a similar manner. The lateral approach is used, splitting the fascia lata longitudinally. The vastus lateralis muscle is carefully detached and retracted anteriorly. The distal femoral metaphysis is exposed without entering the knee joint. The site of insertion of the osteosynthesis plate in the femoral condyle is then prepared. After this the segment of bone to be removed is outlined. The osteotomy is then performed proximally, followed by resection of the femur distally, leaving the medial cortex intact. This results in a wide area of bone contact of the osteotomy fragments which are held in apposition by an osteosynthesis plate (Fig. 1B).

The stability and efficiency of a supracondylar osteotomy is equal to a proximal femoral resection but it has several disadvantages. It is performed close to the knee joint in an area where soft tissue movements are of great importance. Complications of wound healing can result in scar tissue adhesions and may interfere with knee movements. Soft tissue surplus caused by the shortening of bone can create changes in contour of the thigh, resulting in cosmetic deformities. Due to the location of the osteotomy site within the area of free movement of the quadriceps muscle it is possible to lose a certain amount of efficiency of this muscle. This does not happen with intertrochanteric osteotomies. Therefore it is, in general, advisable to employ proximal femoral osteotomies in such cases which require femoral discrepancy correction only. Supracondylar osteotomies are advisable if additional axial correction near the knee joint is necessary.

1 b) Metaphyseal Shortening Osteotomy of the Tibia and Fibula

Shortening osteotomies of the tibia result in cosmetically poorer results than osteotomies of similar dimensions in the femur. This is caused by greater interference with proper limb proportions. It will become even more noticeable if the thigh has its normal length (Fig. 13 c). The knee joint appears to be displaced farther distally resulting in disfigurement. Length of stride becomes noticeably shorter. We recommend considering the indications for this operation very carefully and only rarely shorten the tibia by more than 4 cm. Technically it is possible to shorten the tibia by up to 7 cm if the patient is tall. Proper indications for surgical shortening of the tibia are unilateral pathological elongation caused by increased longitudinal bone growth due to fractures, inflammations or vascular diseases. The operation is performed on the affected limb to accomplish full correction of the discrepancy in length and restitution of normal limb proportions.

The advantage of metaphyseal shortening osteotomies is the rapid bony consolidation of the proximal tibial osteotomy due to the large amount of cancellous bone in the metaphysis.

Operation: Resection of the fibula by the proper amount at the junction of its proximal and middle third. Exposure of the proximal tibial metaphysis by an anterior incision. Delineation of the proximal osteotomy site just below the tibial tubercle. Delineation of the distal osteotomy site by the necessary amount of correction, followed by horizontal resection of the tibia proximally and distally. Apposition of the osteotomy surfaces is followed by fixation with a small angle plate or a T-plate using compression (Fig. 1 C).

Metaphyseal shortening osteotomies have one marked disadvantage. It is difficult to close the incision due to restriction of soft tissue mobility at the proximal third of the tibia. This can lead to wound closure problems. Soft tissue pressure, particularly in the presence of postoperative edema, can damage the deep branch of the peroneal nerve. This operation requires very careful intraoperative technique and postoperative care. The danger of complication is much less in diaphyseal shortening osteotomies of the tibia.

2. Diaphyseal Shortening Osteotomies

The indications for diaphyseal shortening osteotomies are conditions which require longitudinal correction only, without the need for additional axial correction. The advantage of this procedure depends on the use of intramedullary nails which permit early weight bearing. This cannot be accomplished by plate fixation. It is incorrect to state that diaphyseal shortening osteotomies frequently result in rotational deformities. The proper technique in using an intramedullary nail avoids this complication. Step cuts enhance rotatory stability and increase the area of bony contact.

Two variations are available for diaphyseal shortening osteotomies of the femur and tibia. They differ in type of devices used for osteosynthesis, i. e. intramedullary nails or compression plates. If anatomically feasible we prefer the use of intramedullary nails. This method allows early weight bearing after shortening osteotomies. Its use eliminates many biomechanical problems at the site of a transverse osteotomy which is not the case if a compression plate is employed. Biomechanical consequences of instability at the site of shortening osteotomies require a brief discussion. Due to technical ease and in attempting to keep the area of resected bone as small as possible it is advisable to osteotomize transversely or by employing a step cut. A transverse osteotomy can be compared to fractures of the same type. They result in a relatively small area of bony surface. It can only be poorly stablized with a plate which lies on the surface of the bone as compared to the relatively good fixation by an intramedullary nail. The nail withstands abnormal stresses at the osteotomy site better than a plate. Plate fixation is more effective in long diagonal osteotomies, analogous to fractures of this type, but more extensive exposure of bone surfaces and increased technical difficulties make this type of osteotomy generally unadvisable.

Instability at the site of osteotomy results in absorption of bone at the end of the fragments and production of excess callus. The intramedullary nail allows telescoping of the fragments and excess callus is quickly consolidated. A compression plate acts differently. Resorption of bone at the osteotomy sites increases the instability as the bone ends lose contact, resulting in loss of compression applied at the time of the plating. This causes further instability and additional reabsorption of bone. The original function of the compression plate is lost as it only acts as a blocking device, keeping the fragments apart and thus preventing bone healing.

For these reasons we recommend the use of intramedullary nails in all situations where their employment is anatomically feasible. Plates should be used for diaphyseal osteotomies only if the use of an intramedullary nail is contraindicated; for example after osteomyelitis, in the presence of marked congenital or acquired deformities of the long bones or in children or adolescents to avoid damage of an epiphyseal plate by an intramedullary nail.

a) Diaphyseal Femoral Shortening Osteotomy

The advantage of the diaphyseal femoral shortening osteotomy is the place of transection. It is still located in the area of origin of the quadriceps, which then allows early range of motion exercises to prevent limited motion of the knee joint. We recommend removing no more than 6 cm of bone to avoid muscular insufficiency and to still accomodate soft tissue shrinkage. In tall patients it is occasionally permissible to remove a larger segment. The first part of the osteotomy is performed in the same way as for an intramedullary nailing. The tip of the greater trochanter is exposed by an short incision, the medullary cavity is entered at this point and is reamed wide enough to accommodate a heavy intramedullary nail which fits snugly within the cortical walls for a distance of sufficient length. We prefer an open osteotomy for removal of the bony segment from the diaphysis. After a lateral incision at the middle third of the femur has been made, the fascia lata is split longitudinally. The vastus lateralis muscle is detached from the intermuscular septum and the linea aspera, exposing the femoral shaft. The osteotomy site is demarcated proximally and distally at the mid-section of the diaphysis. Longitudinal markings above and below the osteotomies allow satisfactory control of the fragments as far as rotation is concerned. A slow oscillating saw is used to cut straight across or in a step-cut fashion, keeping the saw blade moist by irrigation. Soft tissues are stripped from the linea aspera for a distance of 5 cm at each end of the two fragments, allowing for better soft tissue mobility after femoral shortening. This is followed by co-apting the osteotomy site and by inserting the intermedullary nail from the trochanter major over a guide wire (Fig. 2 A_2).

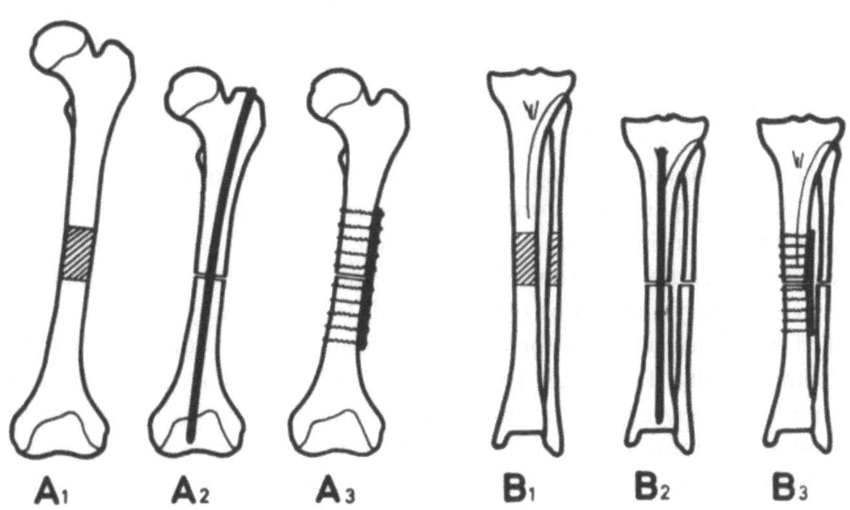

Fig. 2. Diaphyseal shortening osteotomy of femur and tibia (areas of shortening are hatched). A_1 Area of osteotomy for diaphyseal femoral shortening. A_2 Coaptation of fragments and stabilization with intramedullary nail. A_3 Stabilization with compression osteosynthesis plate. B_1 Area of osteotomy for tibia and fibula. B_2 Coaptation of fragments with intramedullary nail. B_3 Stabilization with compression osteosynthesis plate

A diaphyseal osteotomy is rarely ever indicated in infants or adolescents as the presence of an open trochanteric epiphyseal plate prevents entering the medullary cavity from the greater trochanter. This would result in damaging the epiphyseal plate and in developing a valgus deformity of the femoral neck. If such an operation is unavoidable one should enter the medullary cavity through a cortical window distal to the trochanter. A tibial nail is then inserted; its proximal bend (Herzog curvature) has to extend laterally to the cortical window. It is possible to stimulate bone growth by employing an intramedullary nail and by reaming the cavity. This will counteract the lower limb length correction. It is therefore advisable to perform diaphyseal shortening osteotomies in juveniles by employing osteosynthesis plate fixation. This will result in less bone growth stimulation. Metal implants should be removed as soon as consolidation of the osteotomy site has taken place to shorten their growth-stimulating effect as much as possible.

In performing a diaphyseal shortening osteotomy with compression plate fixation it is not necessary to go through the preparatory steps of an intramedullary nailing. The resection of bone corresponding to the amount of shortening required is carried out as described previously. An osteosynthesis plate is applied after the fragments have been co-apted. Screw fixation is first obtained at one end of the osteotomy and, after compression has been applied, at the other end (Fig. 2 A_3).

b) Diaphyseal Shortening Osteotomy of the Tibia

In general the operation is performed in a similar manner as for the femur. First, the necessary amount of bone is removed from the junction of the proximal and middle third of the fibula. Next a longitudinal incision is made proximal to the tibial tuberosity splitting the ligamentum patellae lengthwise. The cortex of the tibia is then broached and the medullary cavity reamed. This is followed by resection of the tibia in its middle third. A step-cut osteotomy will result in better stability against rotation of the fragments and in a larger area of bone apposition (Fig. 2B_1). A snuggly fitting intramedullary nail will stabilize the properly aligned fragments after the leg has been shortened.

Diaphyseal shortening osteotomies have several advantages. Secure fixation with an intermedullary nail can be obtained. Soft tissue mobility is better in the middle third of the leg allowing for better distribution of the soft tissue excess proximally and distally. This facilitates closure. The disadvantage of slower bony consolidation of diaphyseal osteotomies is outweighed by the high tolerance to stress of today's intramedullary nails. Therefore it is better to employ a diaphyseal osteotomy for correction of leg length discrepancies except for such cases which require infracondylar axial correction when a metaphyseal osteotomy should be performed. Compression plate osteosynthesis for diaphyseal leg shortening procedures is indicated in such situations where an intramedullary nail cannot be employed; for example, in anatomical deformities of the tibia, after inflammatory bone changes where intramedullary reaming should be avoided, and in patients with growing bones where an intramedullary nail would result in damage to the epiphyseal plate which could lead to growth deformities.

The operation is limited to resection of the necessary amount of bone from fibula and tibia. The osteotomy site is bridged by an osteosynthesis plate after the fragments have been properly aligned. The plate should be placed against the *lateral* cortex of the tibia. Final fixation is carried out after compression has been applied. Occasionally it is advisable to secure the fibula fragment with a small osteosynthesis plate from the AO small fragment collection.

An anterior compartment syndrome can be avoided if the soft tissues are handled carefully.

B. Operations on a Shortened Lower Limb

Operative Leg Lengthening in One Stage

Operative leg lengthening in one stage depends on the following principles: (1) osteotomy of the involved bone, (2) more or less forceful distraction by mechanical means, (3) preservation of accomplished elongation by osteosynthesis internal fixation, (4) autogenous cancellous bone grafting for bridging purposes or to speed up bony healing at the distraction site. Limited distensibility of the soft tissues and vulnerability of nerves and blood vessels to damage by distraction limit the amount of length which can be gained by such single stage lengthening osteotomies. Experience has shown that a maximum of 4 cm length can be obtained in one stage. For all practical purposes it is restricted to the femur. For anatomical reasons longitudinal distraction of the tibia is accompanied by a high risk factor. Unilateral metaphyseal lengthening osteotomies are indicated in such patients who require correction of alignment of the proximal or distal femoral end and where only a slight amount of lengthening is needed at the same time. Indications for one-stage diaphyseal lengthening osteotomies are conditions which require small amounts of elongation if corrections by conservative means are to be avoided, or where a preceding tibia elongation did not result in full lower limb equalization.

1. Metaphyseal Femoral Lengthening Osteotomy in One Stage

The best indication for such an operation is a valgus deformity of the distal femur with concomitant shortening. A horizontal supracondylar osteotomy leaving the medial cortex intact is performed through a lateral approach. The valgus deformity is corrected by an appropriate open wedge excision. In this manner it is possible to correct axial alignment and to gain some femoral length. The osteotomy site is filled with autogenous cancellous bone after the osteotomy has been stabilized with an angle plate. Relative stability of the osteotomy is guaranteed and bone healing will take place rapidly due to the intact medial cortex opposite the angle plate (Fig. 3).

Different conditions prevail if a varus deformity has to be corrected in the supracondylar femoral region or in rectifying varus or valgus deformities of the femoral neck by intertrochanteric osteotomies. To gain length it is necessary to distract the fragments by osteotomizing the proximal cortex on both sides after the

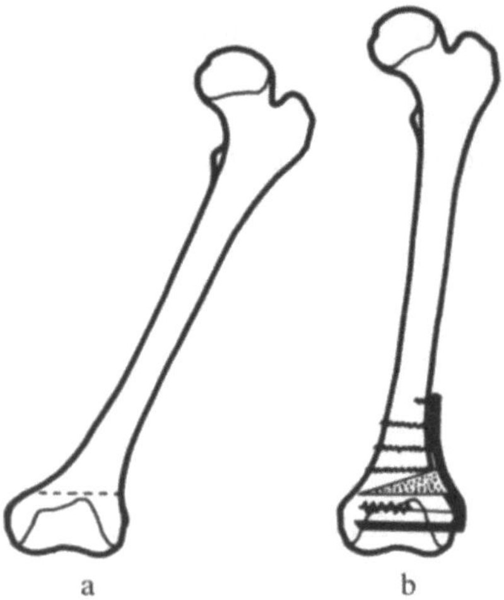

Fig. 3. Metaphyseal lengthening of the distal femur with correction of valgus deformity in one stage (area of autologous spongiosa implantation shaded). (a) Direction of osteotomy starting laterally and leaving medial cortex intact. (b) Valgus deformity is corrected by a lateral opening wedge resulting in gain of some length. The osteotomy site is filled with autologous cancellous bone; the fragments are stabilized by employing an angle plate. The remaining contact of the medial cortex adds to the stability of the osteosynthesis and results in quick bony consolidation

angle plate has been inserted. Pressure of the fragments is exerted solely on the plate, making such osteotomies relatively unstable in spite of carefully filling the gap with autologous spongiosa, and bone healing is delayed. These patients have to be observed carefully during the postoperative period and the indication for this operation is rather limited. A one-stage metaphyseal lengthening osteotomy should be contemplated only if additional axial corrections are required at the proximal or distal femoral end. A diaphyseal lengthening osteotomy is preferable in situations where only a small amount of shortening has to be corrected because conditions for an osteosynthesis are much better in this segment.

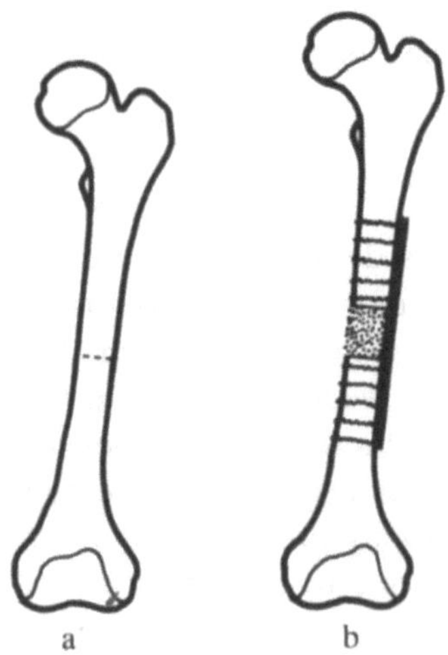

Fig. 4. One-stage diaphyseal femoral lengthening (area of autologous bone graft shaded). (a) Direction of osteotomy in the mid-section of shaft. (b) Distraction of fragments and their fixation with a straight osteosynthesis plate; the area of distraction is filled with an autologous bone graft

2. Diaphyseal Femoral Lengthening In One Stage

Diaphyseal lengthening osteotomies of the femur in one stage are relatively simple operations. A transverse osteotomy is carried out after the diaphysis of the femur has been exposed. An osteosynthesis plate is then fixed to one fragment. The fragments are distracted and the plate is connected to the other fragment. The bony gap is then filled with autologous cancellous bone. The firmness of the cortex and the solidity of a wide long osteosynthesis plate guarantees sufficient stability. The implanted autologous bone graft results in relatively quick bony consolidation. Fixation of a diaphyseal lengthening osteotomy with an intramedullary nail is contraindicated as such a nail requires bony spacers of proper length to keep the fragments apart. It has no advantage compared to an osteotomy plate.

3. Diaphyseal Lengthening Osteotomy With Continuous Distraction (Author's Own Method)[1]

The principle of this operation consists of a transverse osteotomy of the shaft of the long bone at its middle section followed by slow and continuous distraction with an apparatus which employs percutaneous Schanz screws anchored in the proximal and distal metaphysis. The distraction apparatus and its fixation in bone is stable enough to eliminate additional external fixation. The limb can be moved freely and the patient is able to ambulate with Canadian crutches 2 to 3 days postoperatively.

The elongation is carried out by the patient himself by turning a serrated screw connected to a worm gear which distracts the square bars of the apparatus, resulting in a steady increase in distance between the two bony fragments. In this manner it is usually possible to gain 1.5 mm of length per day or 1 cm per week. The fragments are united with an osteosynthesis plate after the required distraction has been accomplished. Radiographs will tell if enough callus is present at the site of elongation and if only a plate is required for stability. If callus formation is delayed it is necessary to graft the site with autologous cancellous bone obtained from the iliac crest. Out-patient care is initiated after the wound has healed. No weight is borne on the affected limb until radiographs show sufficient consolidation to allow first partial and later full weight bearing.

We believe that this operation has several advantages in spite of its relative magnitude. The correction is carried out at the site of deformity, normal anatomical conditions are recreated, and remarkable amounts of lengthening are obtainable. In over 150 limb lengthening operations we have been able to gain a maximum of 220 mm in the lower limb length; 160 mm in the femur, 80 mm in the tibia, and 190 mm in the upper arm.

Correction of lower limb discrepancy alone does not solve the problem of disability for many of our patients. Our examinations have shown that more than

[1] The necessary instruments are produced by Robert Mathys, CH 2544-Bettlach, Switzerland. Distributors: Synthes AG.

half of our patients had additional impairments of form or function in neighboring joints or limbs. They too require corrective measures to make the elongation operation worthwhile.

The most commonly observed concomitant changes include mild deformities, subluxations and dislocations of the hip joint, paralytic or insufficient hip muscles, axial deformities of the femoral or tibial shaft, deformities and contractures of the knee area, abnormal bone growth after injuries of epiphyseal plates, ligamentous injuries of the knee joint, malposition or dislocation of the patella and malalignment, contractures or instability of the foot. Measures to correct these concomitant findings are described in another publication. Here we want only to draw attention to these problems and their necessary correction as an important part in the treatment plan.

a) Femoral Lengthening Osteotomy

The patient is placed in a prone position, two pairs of Schanz screws are inserted, parallel to the knee joint axis through stab wounds, one pair at the distal and one pair at the proximal femoral metaphysis. Image intensifier control is helpful for proper orientation of the screws. The shaft of the femur is exposed by a posterolateral approach. The skin incision is carried out laterally at a distance of approximately 5 to 7 cm from the mid-line of the thigh. The space between the musculus vastus lateralis and musculus biceps femoris is bluntly separated. The femoral shaft with its periosteum is osteotomized transversely at the mid-point between the two pairs of Schanz screws. The osteotomy site is drained. The wound is

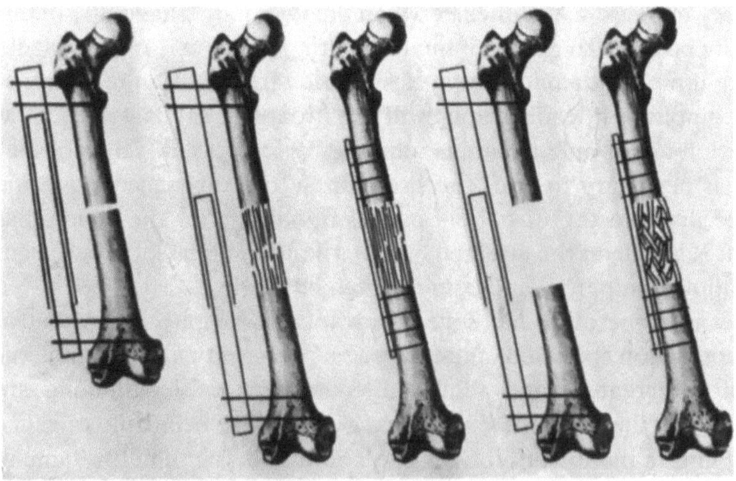

Fig. 5. Femoral lengthening employing continous distraction. (a) Osteotomy accomplished, distraction apparatus in place. (b) and (c) Stabilizing osteosynthesis at conclusion of distraction period and removal of distraction apparatus in the presence of sufficient callus. (d) and (e) Internal fixation, autologous bone grafting (cancellous strips) and removal of distraction apparatus in the absence of sufficient callus (from Chirurg *42,* No. 6, 1971)

closed and a sterile dressing is applied. The distraction apparatus is connected to the Schanz screws and extended by 5 to 6 mm to avoid painful contact between the bone fragments. The resulting soft tissue tension helps to stabilize the traction apparatus. Postoperative elongation is controlled by the patient. The soft tissue channels around the Schanz screws are carefully observed and cared for. Physical therapy is mainly directed toward knee motion and safe ambulation with Canadian crutches without weight bearing on the involved extremity. Occasionally it is necessary to lengthen the knee flexors or to perform an adductor tenotomy if soft tissues are rigid or if a large amount of lengthening is required. This is done while the distraction apparatus is still in place.

X-rays are taken after the necessary length has been obtained. This will tell if enough callus has formed at the elongation site or if autologous bone graft will be neccessary at the time of osteosynthesis. The Schanz screws may bend due to soft tissue tension if a large amount of lengthening is necessary. This can result in a varus deviation of the fragments. Correction of this deviation is accomplished under X-ray control by realigning the screws in their anchorage to the distraction apparatus.

The osteosynthesis at the end of the lengthening process is carried out with the patient prone and the distraction apparatus in place. The previous incision is utilized to expose the femoral shaft and the fragments are connected with a wide sturdy osteosynthesis plate. Strips of cancellous bone obtained from the posterior iliac crest are inserted in the absence of sufficient callus formation. The distraction apparatus is removed after the wound has been closed.

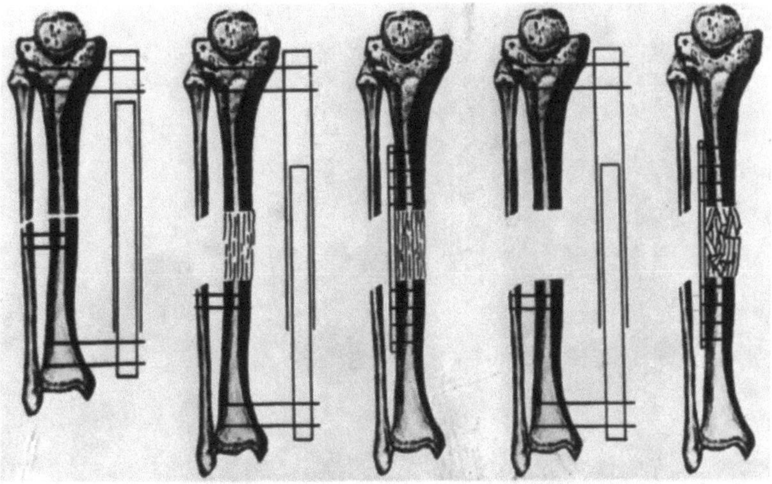

a b c d e

Fig. 6. Leg lengthening employing continuous distraction. (a) Oblique osteotomy of fibula and transverse osteotomy of tibia accomplished, distal fibular fragment connected with the tibia by two fixation screws, distraction apparatus in place. (b) and (c) Stabilizing internal fixation and removal of distraction apparatus at end of the distraction period in presence of adequate callus formation. (d) and (e) Stabilizing internal fixation, cancellous bone graft at site of distraction in absence of adequate callus formation and removal of distraction apparatus (from Chirurg *42,* No. 6, 1971)

b) Lengthening Osteotomy of the Tibia

The operation is performed with the patient supine. First it is necessary to protect the ankle joint by connecting the distal fibula with the tibia to avoid proximal migration of the lateral malleolus caused by the pull of the soft tissues during the lengthening process. From a lateral skin incision the fibula is exposed at the junction of its middle and lower portion and the lateral aspect of the tibia is exposed along the interosseous membrane. Two cortical screws are then inserted, penetrating all four cortices, thus preventing movement of the two bones against each other. The fibula is transected proximal to the fixation screws.

The next step is the insertion of two pairs of Schanz screws parallel to the knee joint axis into the proximal and distal tibial metaphysis through medial stab incisions. Following this, the tibia with its periosteum is osteotomized transversely at the mid-point between the two pairs of screws through an anterior approach. The wound is then drained, closed, and protected by a sterile dressing. The application of the distraction apparatus medially is the last step of the operation. Postoperative care is similar to that employed in femoral continuous lengthening procedures. An Achilles tenotomy with the distraction apparatus in

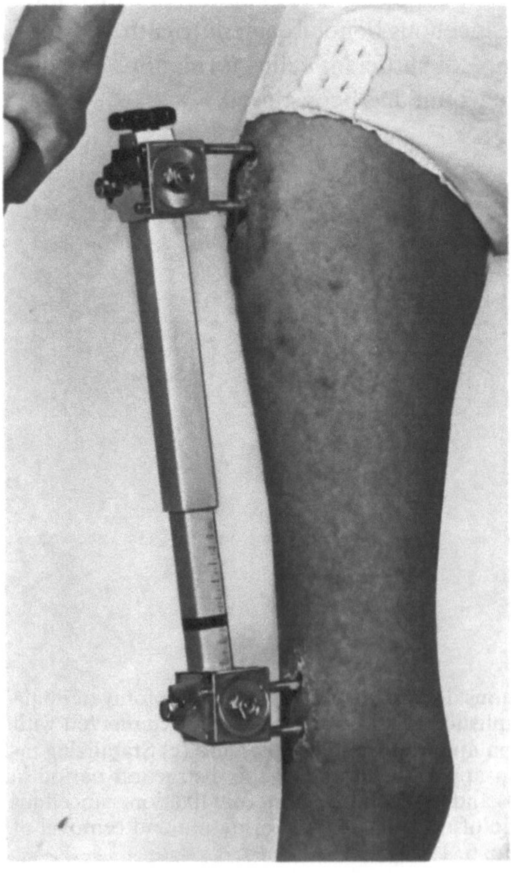

Fig. 7. Female 16 years old (status after poliomyelitis). Femoral lengthening operation. Position of distraction apparatus at lateral aspect of the thigh (from Chirurg. *42,* No. 6, 1971)

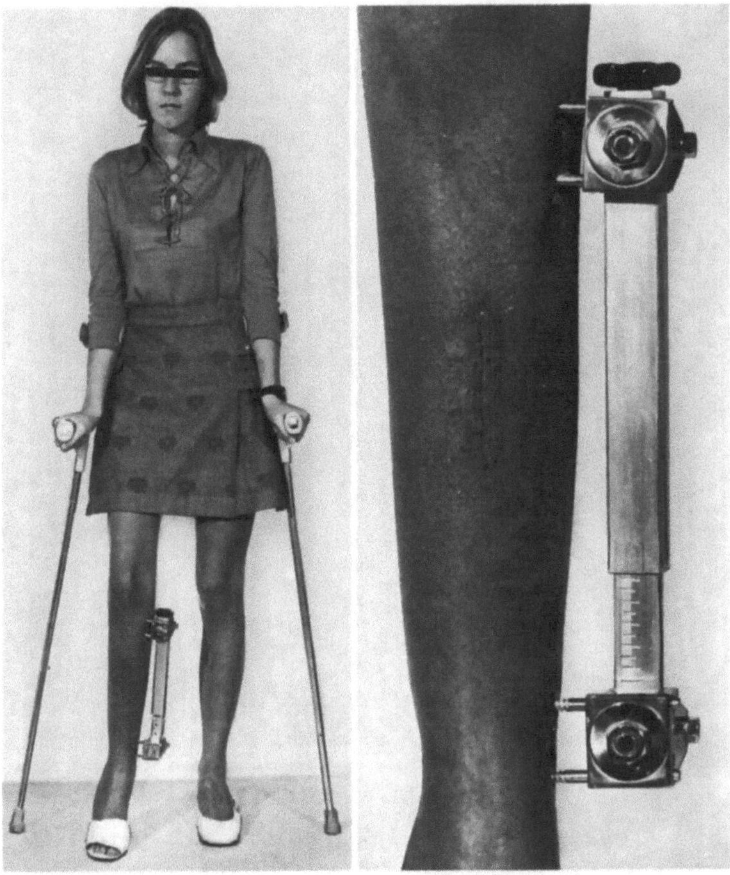

Fig. 8. Female 19 years of age, congenital leg shortening. Tibial lengthening operation. Position of distraction apparatus at medial aspect of leg (from Chirurg *42*, No. 6, 1971)

place to avoid equinus contracture of the foot is performed, if a large amount of length has to be gained. Soft tissue tension of the calf muscles can result in bending of the Schanz screws leading to anterior bowing of the tibia fragments. This can cause pressure and damage of the overlying skin. It can be prevented by realigning the Schanz screws in the opposite direction at their connection to the distraction apparatus.

At the conclusion of the elongation period the tibia is exposed by an incision of 4 mm lateral to the anterior tibial border. The distraction site is bridged with a thin osteosynthesis plate which is placed against the lateral cortex of the tibia. If necessary, autologous cancellous bone obtained from the inner aspect of the anterior iliac crest is placed into the area of lengthening. The distraction apparatus is removed after wound closure. The patient is discharged home after the wound has healed, using Canadian crutches for ambulation.

Indications for surgical intervention are conditions in which the patient can expect a marked improvement of his disability. The amount of leg length disa b c d

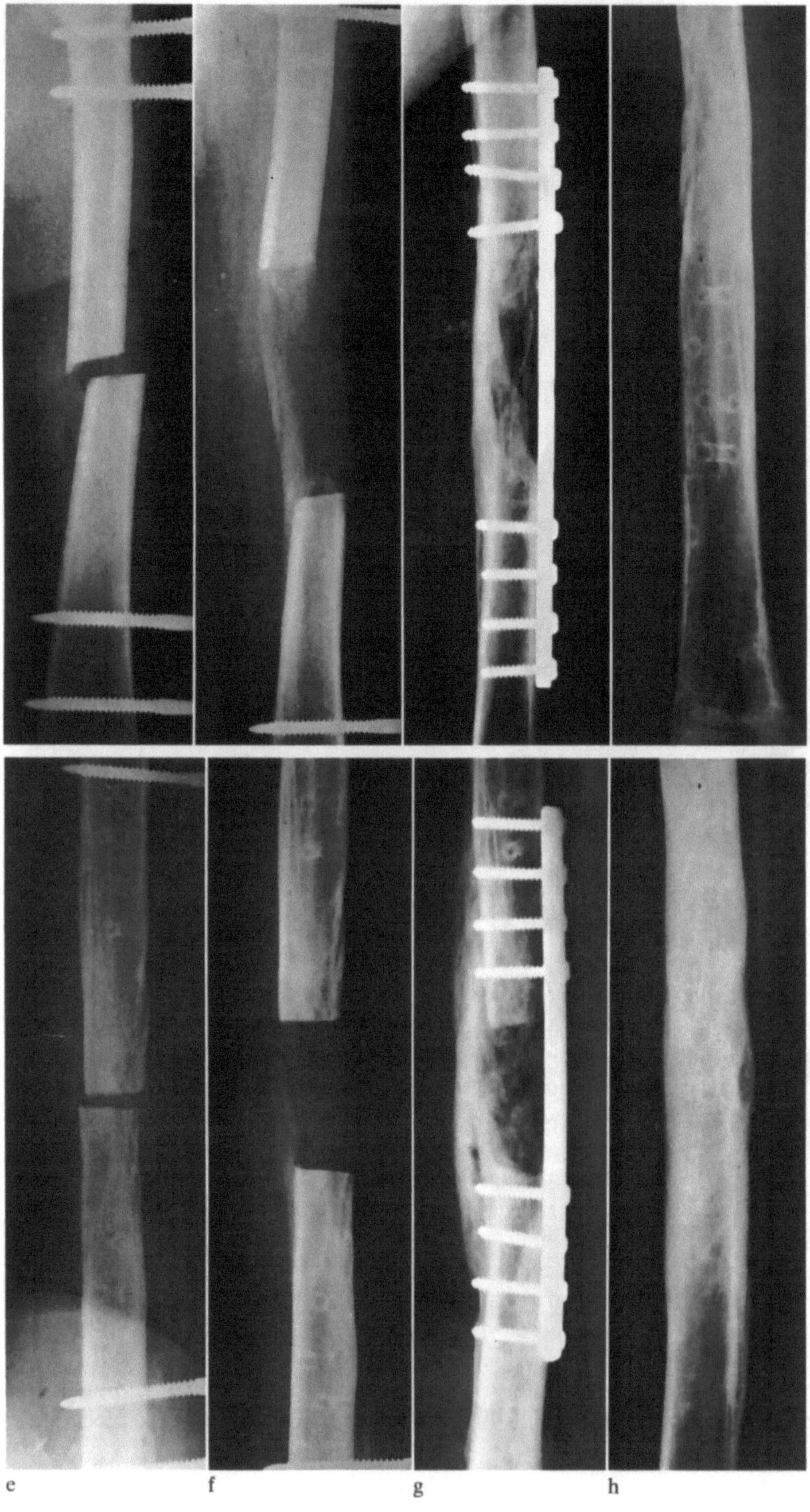

e f g h

Fig. 9

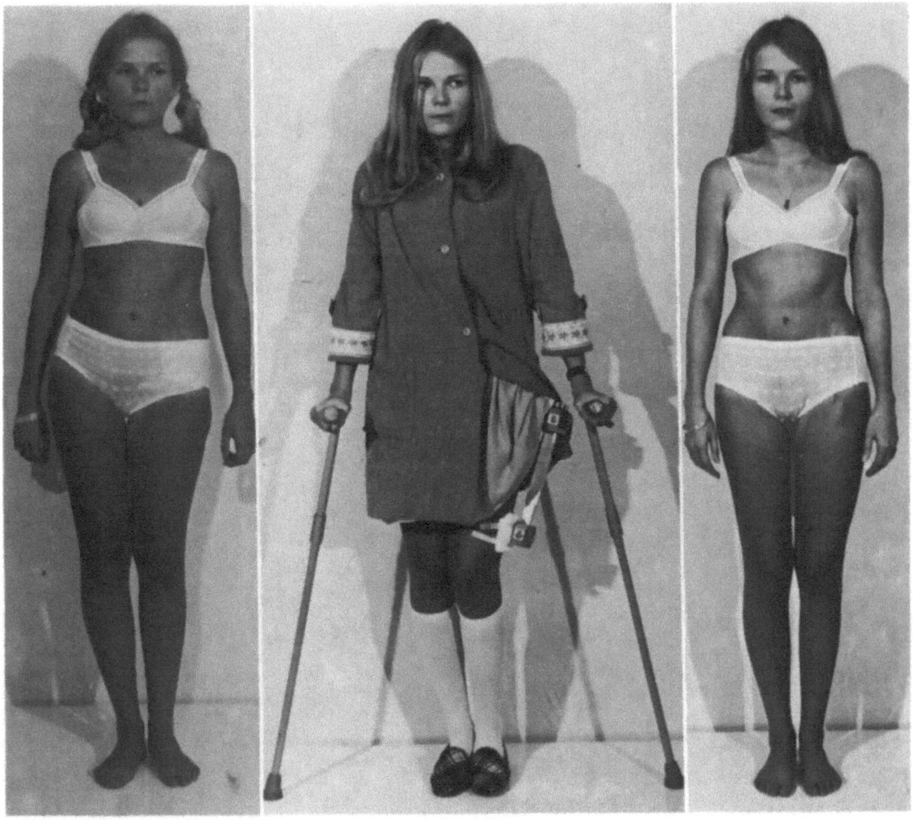

a b c

Fig. 10. A 16-year-old female; status after conservative treatment of congenital dislocation of the left hip resulting in 5 cm shortening. (a) Before, (b) during, and (c) 4 months after left femoral osteotomy with full equalization of lower limb length

Fig. 9. (a) Left femoral shortening of 7 cm as a result of coxitis, girl 10 years old; lengthening osteotomy; distraction apparatus in place. (b) Ten weeks later, femoral lengthening of 9.5 cm overcorrection of 2.5 cm, minimal callus formation. (c) Bony consolidation medially, 5 months after osteosynthesis and cancellous bone grafting. (d) Bony consolidation of entire distraction area and extensive remodeling of medullary cavity, $2^1/_2$ years after surgery. In the meantime recurrent femoral shortening of 5 cm caused by growth spurt. (e) Reosteotomy and lengthening at previous operative site. (f) Gain of 5 cm length, no callus, 4 weeks postoperatively. (g) Bony consolidation medially, 14 weeks after osteosynthesis and bone grafting. (h) Three years after osteosynthesis and bone grafting

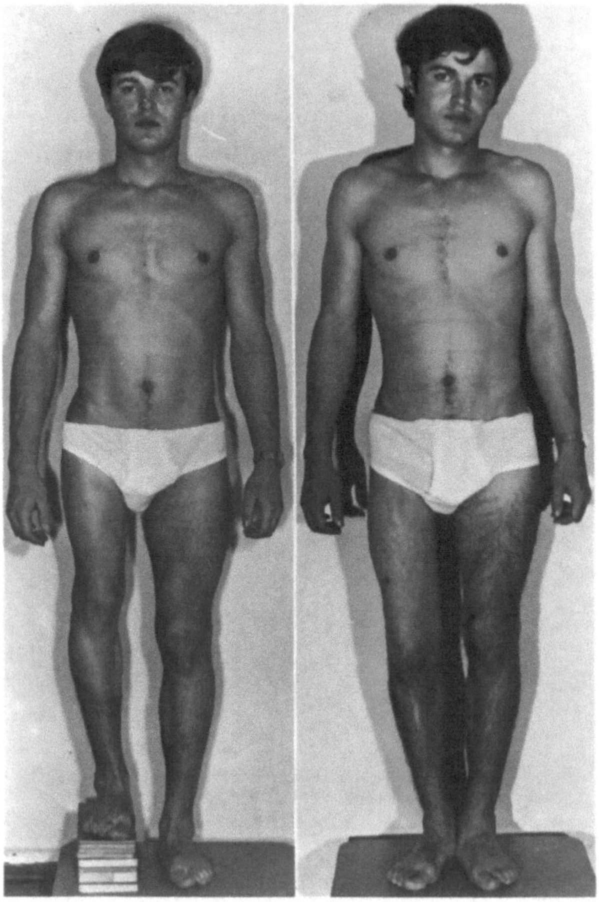

a b

Fig. 11. (a) A 10 cm thigh shortening, right, in a male aged 18, as a result of coxitis. (b) One year after lengthening osteotomy of the right femur with complete correction. Marked normalization of the muscles of the right lower limb

crepancy should be 4 cm or more, and the state of the soft tissues should allow complete correction or, in the case of extreme shortening, at least assure a residual amount of shortening of no more than 3 cm. Additional stabilizing and corrective measures in treating the concomitant deformities should free the patient from major orthotic devices. The described operation is contraindicated if the patient will have to wear a large orthopaedic apparatus *after* such lengthening procedures as it is easily possible to correct any amount of limb shortening with these external aids.

Indications for Operative Lower Limb Discrepancy Corrections

The previously mentioned and explained methods for correction of leg length discrepancies show that we have many choices and reliable operations to correct them. The individual methods are based on different principles. They have exactly defined advantages and disadvantages and are clearly limited in their indication. They represent a wide therapeutic spectrum for the treatment of an important disability. Remarkable amounts of lower limb length discrepancies can be accurately corrected by one or the other method.

It remains the duty of the physician to select the proper operation or combination of operations to obtain the optimum result even with these significant advances in surgical techniques. He has to consider every possible individual factor before he decides to operate. The rational evaluation of *all* problems arising

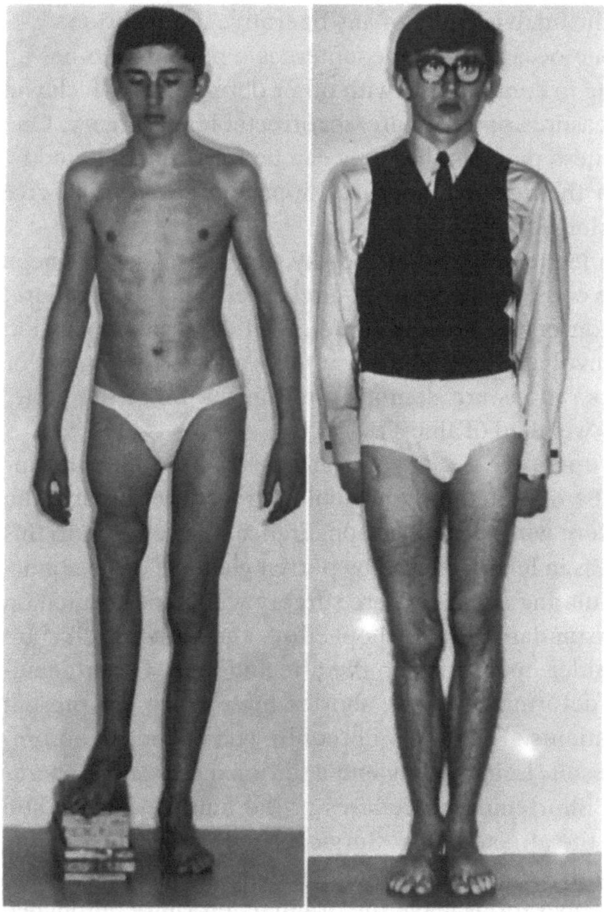

a b

Fig. 12. (a) A 20 cm lower limb shortening right, in a male aged 15, as a result of osteomyelitis during infancy. (b) Result after 15 cm femoral and 5 cm tibial lengthening, right; correction of pes equinus and knee joint revision, right. The patient walks without a limp and for unlimited distances in regular shoes from the patient's disability, and an understanding of the reliability, magnitude and risk of all technical or surgical methods for the correction of leg length discrepancies are prerequisites if we are to properly advise the patient of the best possible treatment program for his individual disability. It is totally wrong to dogmatically accept only one operation as the proper method, as the previously mentioned operations are of equal value. The patient has the right to be informed of all possibilities and the orthopaedist should be familiar with all methods which might improve these deformities. Careful deliberation of all the possibilities remains the key to proper treatment.

As a first step in outlining a treatment plan one has to consider the basic question of whether conservative means will result in satisfactory correction. Apparently for psychological reasons, it is not uncommon to have patients insist on surgical correction of differences of 1 to 2 cm. The first consultation should settle this desire once and for all by rationally explaining the possibilities of conservative correction and the inadvisability of any operative intervention.

Another problem which one occasionally encounters is a patient who has an extreme amount of shortening in combination with other deformities, which will require extensive surgical measures or which are uncorrectable by surgery. One should never raise hopes in these patients that they can be fully rehabilitated by an operation and explain to them that modern orthopaedic devices will give them a better chance to function adequately.

If the decision to correct a leg length discrepancy by surgical means has been made, it becomes necessary to consider the value of a relatively simple procedure, such as a shortening operation of the healthy limb, or an extensive operation such as a lengthening of the involved limb. The advantages and disadvantages of shortening or lengthening operations are demonstrated in the following table. They will have to be carefully weighed (Table 1).

One major advantage of operative leg lengthening is the fact that the involved, "crippled limb" will be operated on. Shortening procedures involve the intact healthy limb and interfere with its normal appearance. (Exceptions to this are cases of pathological excess in length caused by partial giantism or by abnormal bone growth due to stimulating agents, where surgery will be performed on the affected side.) It is understandable that orthopaedists and patients alike are more readily inclined to consider operations on the affected limb. Other deciding factors are concomitant deformities of the shorter limb which are present in more than half of these patients. They too will require corrections to accomplish an optimal functional result. Lengthening and additional corrective operations involve the same limb. Shortening procedures of the uninvolved side still require corrective surgery of the affected limb. Surgical lengthening corrects the lower limb deformity directly. It can result in obtaining the complete restoration of a normal limb. Shortening operations leave the original deformity untouched resulting only in a compensating mechanism of the healthy limb. To some extent they cause a symmetrical duplication of the deformity. This is of great importance in regard to body height and body proportions. Lower limb lengthening preserves body height, lower limb shortening reduces it. This consideration is

Table 1. Indications for surgical shortening or lengthening in leg length discrepancy. Comparison of advantages (+) and disadvantages (−) of surgical shortening or lengthening

Leg lengthening	Leg shortening
+ Surgery on the affected limb	− Operation of the uninvolved limb
+ Correction of concomitant deformities of the involved limb	− Operation on both legs necessary if concomitant deformities have to be corrected
+ Correction of deformity (restitutio ad integrum)	− Compensation of deformity
+ Preservation of body length	− Diminution of body height
+ Normalization of body proportions	− Interference with body proportions
+ Can be done on femur and/or tibia	− Leg operations may lead to complications
+ Gain of length up to 22 cm	− Limitation of correction up to approximately 10 cm
+ Shortening of uninvolved limb usually not necessary	− Lengthening of the shortened limb frequently necessary
− Long hospitalization (6 weeks–6 months)	+ Short hospitalization (3 weeks)
− Slow consolidation (8 weeks–8 months)	+ Quick bony consolidation (8–12 weeks)
− Cancellous grafting frequently necessary	+ No cancellous bone graft at osteotomy site
− Increasing problems with advancing age	+ Age of no importance
− Operation technically difficult	+ Operation technically easy
− Three- to four-stage surgery necessary (osteotomy, osteosynthesis, spongiosa grafting, metallic implant removal)	+ Two-stage operation (osteotomy, removal of metallic implants)
− Concomitant surgery frequently necessary (achillotenotomy, knee flexor lengthening)	+ No concomitant surgery required
− Temporary restriction of motion of adjacent joints caused by soft tissue tension	+ No restriction of joint motion

relatively unimportant in tall patients. Smaller patients in general are not willing to undergo a shortening osteotomy which will result in further diminution of their height. Preservation of proper body proportions is extremely important in corrections of larger amounts of lower limb discrepancies. Operative lower limb lengthening restores normal body proportions as it is performed at the site of deformity. Shortening of the healthy limb will result in disturbance of body proportions and therefore creates additional aesthetic problems. This has to be considered carefully in female patients. Composite photography represents this phenomenon strikingly (Figs. 13 and 14). Shortening of the lower extremities causes the impression of excessive length of the torso and the upper limbs.

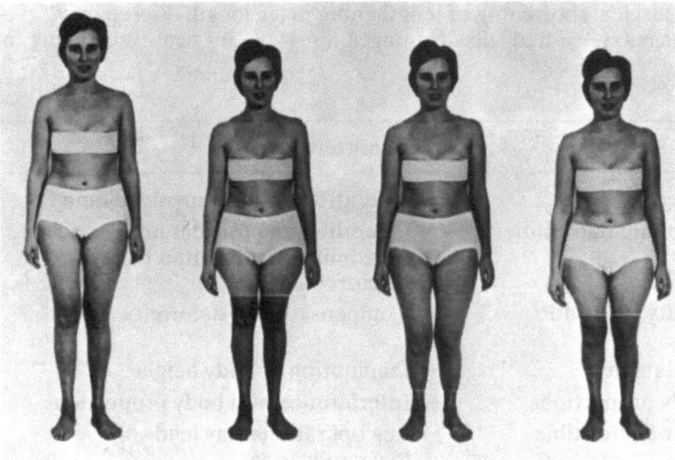

a b c d

Fig. 13. Composite photograph to demonstrate body proportions. (a) Female, 26 years old with normal body proportions. (b) Composite picture showing a shortening of both femora by 7.5 cm. (e) Composite picture showing shortening of both tibiae by 7.5 cm. (d) Composite picture showing shortening of femora and tibiae by 5 cm each. Composite photographs show marked disfiguration of large amounts of lower limb shortening in regard to body proportions

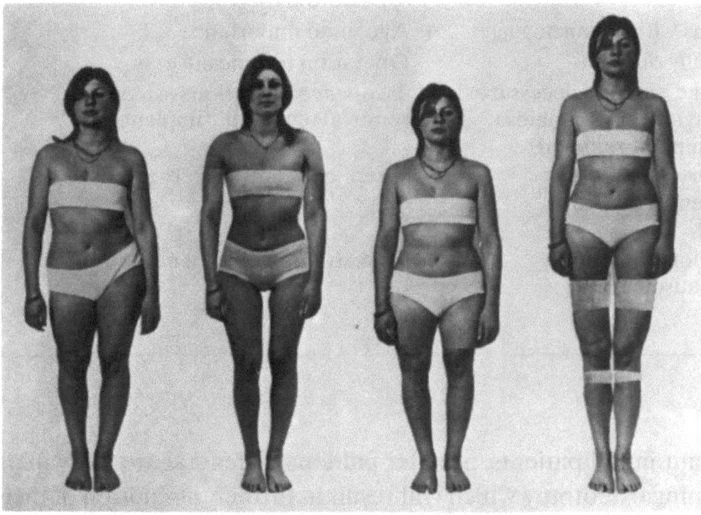

a b c d

Fig. 14. Composite photograph to demonstrate body proportions. (a) Female, 24 years old, with marked shortening of right lower limb as a result of right-sided hip joint sepsis during infancy, with shortening and varus deformity of the left knee joint following Blount epiphyseodesis of the distal left femur and proximal left tibia; residual shortening of the right femur of 8.5 cm. (b) Result of operative lengthening of the right femur by 8.5 cm (unretouched photograph). (c) Composite picture showing the results if shortening of the left femur by 8.5 cm had been carried out. (d) Composite picture showing the results if epiphyseodesis had not been performed and total lower limb discrepancy had been treated by full correction of the inequality by a lengthening operation

Shortening of the thighs in the presence of normal leg length and even more so shortening of the legs in the presence of normal thigh length are felt to be particularly deforming. This aesthetic problem alone limits the feasible amount of shortening in osteotomies for lower limb equalization. Surgical lengthening can be performed by operations of similar magnitude on either femur or the tibia. Operative shortening has its main indication in surgery involving the femur. It is much more problematic if performed in the tibia. There is also a quantitative difference between these operations. It is technically possible to lenghten a limb by amounts up to 22 cm; aesthetic reasons, soft tissue excess and muscular insufficiencies limit shortening operations to 10 cm. Consequently, it is possible to completely correct leg length discrepancies by surgical lengthening in most instances. It is seldom necessary to achieve further correction by additional shortening of the other limb. Lower limb equalization by shortening frequently requires additional lengthening of the involved side, particularly in cases with marked discrepancies.

The advantages of lengthening operations have to be weighed against several serious disadvantages inherent in this procedure.

Of particular importance is the length of hospitalization. Depending on the amount of inequality, in-patient care may require 6 weeks to 6 months as compared to approximately 3 weeks of hospitalization required for shortening procedures. Bony consolidation of lengthening operations takes 8 weeks to 8 months; patients with shortening osteotomies usually start full weight bearing after 8 to 12 weeks. The majority of patients with lengthening osteotomies need autologous cancellous bone grafting. They are never required in shortening operations.

Successful results with lengthening operations become more difficult in patients over 20 years of age, as the soft tissues lose their elasticity after this time. In addition, the osteotomy no longer heals as readily. Lengthening osteotomies after the age of 40 are contraindicated. Shortening osteotomies on the other hand can be performed regardless of the patient's age.

Lengthening osteotomies are technically difficult to perform; shortening osteotomies are generally easy procedures. Lengthening requires three to four stages (osteotomy, osteosynthesis, cancellous bone graft, removal of metallic implants); shortening is carried out in two stages (osteotomy, removal of metallic implants). Additional surgery is frequently needed in lengthening operations (achillotenotomy, adductor tenotomy, knee flexor lengthening.) They are not required in shortening operations. Soft tissue tension frequently results in temporary restriction of motion of the adjacent joints in patients who have undergone lengthening procedures, in contrast to shortening osteotomies, which may occasionally develop muscular insufficiencies but no restriction of motion.

Summary

Several effective but basically dissimilar operations are available for the correction of lower limb discrepancies. While the variety of choices makes the appropriate selection more difficult, it also permits the selection of the proper combination which will be right in any given situation. The careful evaluation of the lower leg length discrepancy as it affects the patient and the careful consideration of the effectiveness of corrective measures will help to decide which approach should be recommended. One should recognize that very severe lower limb discrepancies cannot be treated surgically. They require efficient orthopaedic mechanical devices to improve the functional capabilities of these patients.

References

Anderson, W. V.: J. Bone Jt Surg. **34 B,** 150 (1952).
Fischer, S.: Die Rehabilitation **8,** 147 (1969).
Fischer, S.: Ärztl. Mitteil. **67,** 2523 (1970).
Küntscher, G.: Z. Orthop. **98,** 123 (1964).
Morscher, E., Taillard, W.: Beinlängenunterschiede. Basel-New York: S. Karger 1965.
Müller, M. E., Allgöwer, M., Willenegger, H.: Manual der Osteosynthese – AO-Technik. Berlin-Heidelberg-New York: Springer 1969.
Wagner, H.: Chirurg **42,** 260 (1971).

English translation from the German edition *Der Orthopäde,* Vol. 1, pp. 59–74 (1972),

The Injured Knee

The Importance of Arthrography Following Trauma to the Knee Joint

A. Rüttimann and Ch. Kieser*

Timing of Arthrography

In the absence of compelling arguments to the contrary, arthrography should wait several weeks after a fresh trauma, i.e., until the hemarthrosis is resorbed and a good view of the interior of the joint is guaranteed. This holds especially true for fresh meniscus lesions combined with injury to the collateral ligament, where the diagnosis is not always clear.

Thus, arthrography in fresh trauma is rare. Coagulated blood can cause difficulties in localization and diagnosis, cover up pathologic findings or simulate free-floating bodies.

Plain Roentgenogram

The second prerequisite for successful arthrography is suitable plain roentgenograms of the knee joint.

The type and number of films depend on the case in question. In every post-traumatic state, generally in equivocal knee complaints and also when a meniscus lesion is suspected, conventional a-p and lateral roentgenograms are absolutely necessary. Additional bone injuries, even minor ones, and other bony abnormalities (dysplasias, inflammations, tumors, chondropathies, osteochondropathies, chondrocalcinoses, etc.) can thereby be excluded. A positive Rauber's sign (an osteophyte on the medial border of the tibial plateau) can indicate a preexisting or old meniscus lesion. The plain roentgenogram is the indispensable document for subsequent expert medical opinion.

In questions of stability a-p films of the knee joint held in moderate flexion are indicated. For films in adduction, a balloon or pillow is placed between the knees; the ankles are tied together in elastic traction. Or, vice versa, the balloon can be placed between the ankles and the knee held together with tape above the joint.

* Institut für Röntgendiagnostik und Chirurgische Klinik, Stadtspital Triemli, Zurich, Switzerland

These examinations of stability are contraindicated during the healing phase of collateral ligament lesions, but rather should be done directly following the injury (same day) or after 8–10 weeks have passed. In forced adduction or abduction an "air" arthrogram may be produced, in which case the meniscus and the contours of the cartilage can be visualized. However, this is not sufficient for a satisfactory evaluation of the internal structures of the knee.

In addition, films taken with the knee held in the drawer position are practicable for assessment of cruciate ligament function. If it is a question of overloading in the area of the knee joint, then obviously views of the neighboring joints, above all the hip joint, the pelvis, and if necessary the spine, and the remaining bones are essential.

If the standard films suggest "wear and tear" changes in the cartilage, this may be confirmed by an a-p standing film.

In unicompartmental cartilage destruction the joint space may show no corresponding narrowing in the X-ray taken with the patient in the supine position, whereas in the standing position it may be clearly manifest.

For evaluation of the patella axial films are essential.

In certain cases spot-film procedures are necessary: A bone lesion of minimal extent may be so situated that conventional radiography is of no avail. Here, spot fluoroscopy of the suspicious areas is worthwhile, e.g., in serial films taken tangential to a pressure-sensitive site, taking care to choose the most appropriate projection. Cup-shaped splinterings on the femoral condyle, for example, or on the patella, may be visualized with tangential plus axial films of the femoropatellar joint.

Tears of the cruciate ligaments are seen better in tunnel films, as are osteochondroses. Other doubtful findings may be elucidated by tomography. The results of roentgen investigations preceding arthrography – and the multifold possibilities presented – are only of use if the radiologist receives beforehand from the orthopaedist specific orientation as to the problem and certain tentative indications, according to which he may proceed selectively in the event that conventional radiography reveals nothing.

Arthrography

There are various methods of arthrography:

1. Air-filling of the knee joint (pneumoarthrography)
2. Filling with liquid, water-soluble contrast medium (positive arthrography)
3. A combination of both methods (double-contrast arthrography)

We have practiced all three methods, especially studies with liquid contrast media, but since 1954 we have changed over to double-contrast methods, which seem to us to produce the most easily interpreted images and are therefore favored by nonradiologists. Of course, we begin all investigations concerning a free-floating body or cartilage damage or other nonmeniscus lesion with air arthrography and then go on to double-contrast methods, mainly in evaluations of the meniscus. Our experiences are based on more than 10,000 investigations performed to date.

Generally, however, the choice of method must be left to the investigator. The best results are achieved by one's own methods. The salient point is not the method but the technical execution and interpretation.

Technique of Investigation (for details, see References)

Following aseptic technique, and under local anesthesia, the needle is introduced into the joint from a lateral position somewhat distal to the upper border of the patella. Existing hemarthroses must first be completely aspirated. The better the emptying of the joint, the better the visualization of the internal structures. We introduce 20–30 cm^3 air in the joint depending on size together with about 3 cm^3 of contrast medium. After removing the needle, some moderate, passive flexion and rotation movements in the standing position serve to distribute the contrast medium. The latter spreads a thin film uniformly over the internal surfaces. Tears in the capsule and menisci and cartilage changes thus may be visualized.

Roentgen Equipment

A good roentgen installation is a prerequisite. The knee is X-rayed and the internal structures selectively visualized, especially the menisci, after which spot films are taken in fixed positions and from different angles of rotation.

Best results are achieved with fluoroscopic apparatus, similar to its use in gastrointestinal studies. An above-table tube, which can be shifted and positioned obliquely (Fig. 1), improves the technique. The knee is held freely in a suitable position in a wooden rack.

The Arthrogram

Arthrography allows a comprehensive evaluation of the whole interior of the joint, not only the meniscus.

Lateral films of the whole joint in medium flexion give a good survey of the internal structures. In addition, the synovial space, the articular cartilage lining, the cruciate ligaments, and the infrapatellar fat pad may be evaluated. Depending upon the findings, additional a-p or oblique projections may be taken.

The patellar cartilage is examined in the lateral and axial projection.

The normal meniscus presents itself as a wedge-shaped, soft-tissue density (transverse view) covered by a thin film of contrast material. The air introduced into the joint delineates the meniscus from the adjacent cartilage which in turn

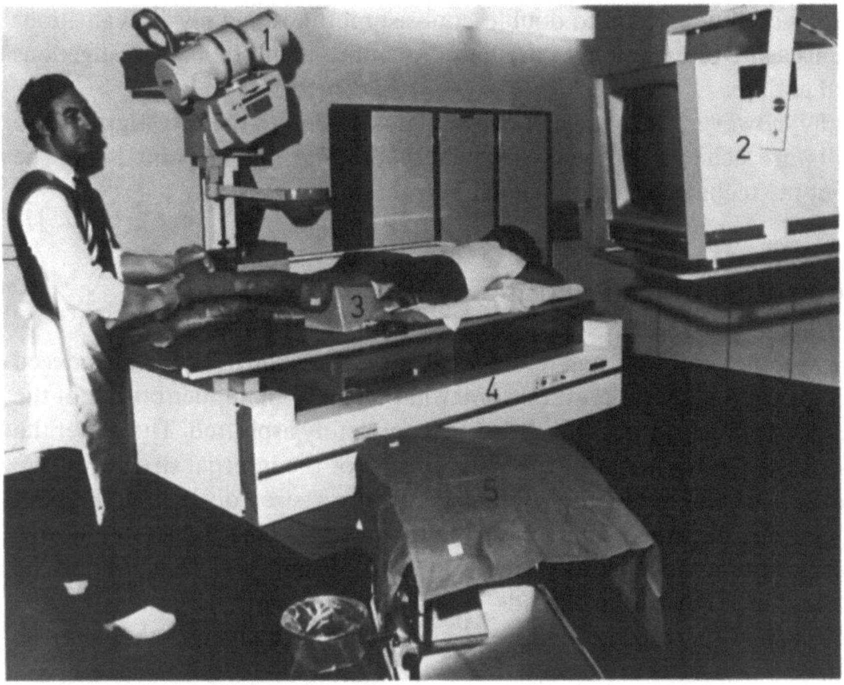

Fig. 1. Roentgen equipment for arthrography. *1* Tube above table, on a swivel for linear tomography. *2* Television apparatus. *3* Wooden block for holding the upper leg in position. *4* Tilting table. *5* Instrument table

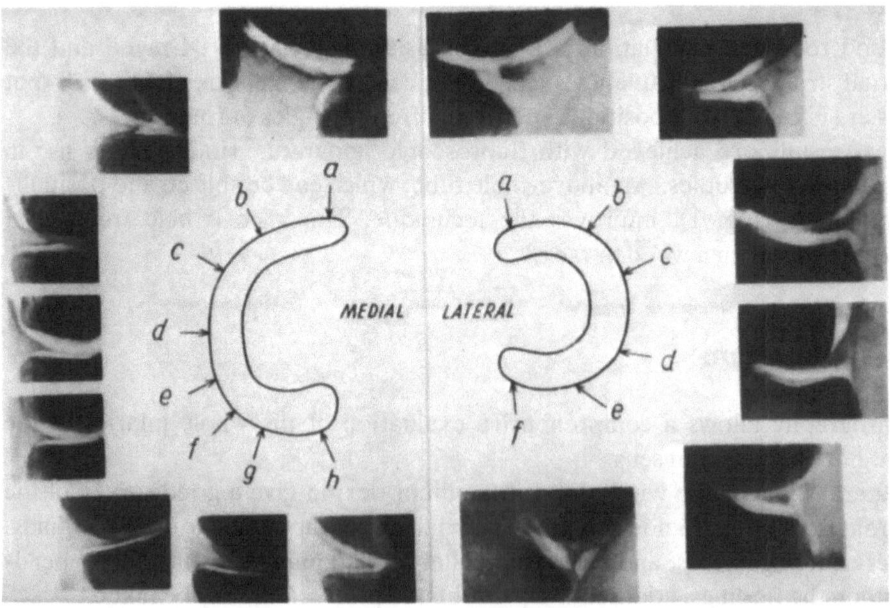

Fig. 2. A general arthrogram of the medial and lateral meniscus. Of the medial meniscus *(left)* eight films *(a–h)* from anterior to posterior horn are presented. Of the lateral meniscus *(right)* six films are shown. *Middle:* Drawings of the two menisci. Arrows designate the parts of the meniscus which correspond to the adjacent arthrograms. (For details, see text)

may be distinguished from the subchondral bone. Eight to twelve pictures of the whole meniscus taken equidistantly allow for a good evaluation of even minor lesions (Fig. 2).

Meniscus tears appear as clefts or deformations in the body of the meniscus. Small discontinuities in the contour of the wedge-shaped meniscus often may signify unimportant lesions. Degenerative changes appear in the form of a swelling of the body of the meniscus and imbibition of liquid contrast medium. Old lesions are likewise differentiated from fresh ones through the marked imbibition at their borders.

Indications for Arthrography

1. *Vague knee complaints with or without a history of trauma,* especially when there are striking differences between the clinical findings and the subjective statements of the patient, or with joint effusions or hemarthroses recurring over a longer period of time, when clinical studies and conventional radiography offer no further clues.
2. *Meniscus injuries,* when the localization of the lesion (lateral or medial) is ambiguous, or in case special operations on the meniscus, as for example, partial resection, are planned.
3. *Post-meniscectomy status,* in the event that long-lasting postoperative complaints persist or if preoperative complaints continue unchanged following the operation.
4. *Expert opinion* in cases where doubt exists as to the role of a preceding operation or the complaints cannot otherwise be clarified.
5. *Old knee joint fractures* causing long-term complaints and in which simultaneous meniscus injuries are present.
6. *Subluxation* or *other patella lesions,* to exclude a meniscus lesion (lateral), since the differential diagnosis is often difficult.
7. In *osteochondral lesions,* for evaluation of the operative procedure and postoperative evaluation of the healing process.
8. *Exact localization of loose bodies in the joints* and in chondromatoses, for complete understanding of the chondroma before operation.

Vague Knee Complaints

G. G., 25-year-old auto mechanic:

Unable to work for one month because of prepatellar medial and anterolateral knee pain. No history of trauma. Pain on pressure in the area of a slightly swollen prepatellar bursa. Mild loss of flexion of about 30°. The knee was initially markedly swollen. Aspiration revealed a hemarthrosis (20 cc) of unclear origin.

Plain film: Slight gonarthrosis.

Arthrogram: Slight rolling out of the posterior horn of the medial meniscus with medium-grade degenerative changes, which, however, do not explain the clinical findings. The suprapatellar pouch (Fig. 3), on the other hand, shows an irregular papillary-villous, roughened posterior wall. The finding corresponds to a typical *pigmented villonodular synovitis,* which was confirmed at operation.

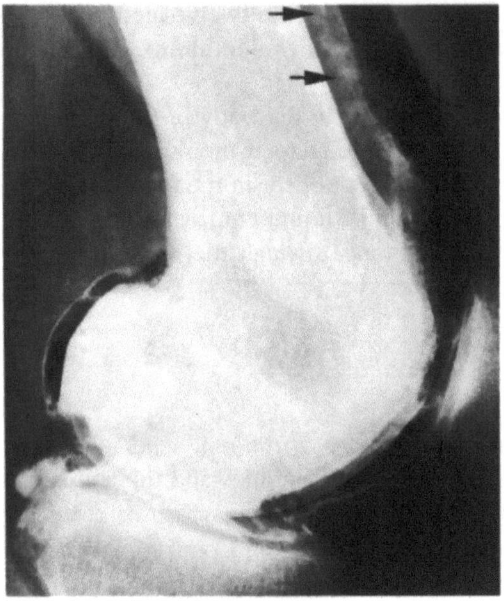

Fig. 3. Double contrast arthrogram of the knee joint. Lateral view. The dorsal wall of the suprapatellar pouch *(arrows)* exhibits an irregular, nodular, bulbous quality: Dx: pigmented villonodular synovitis

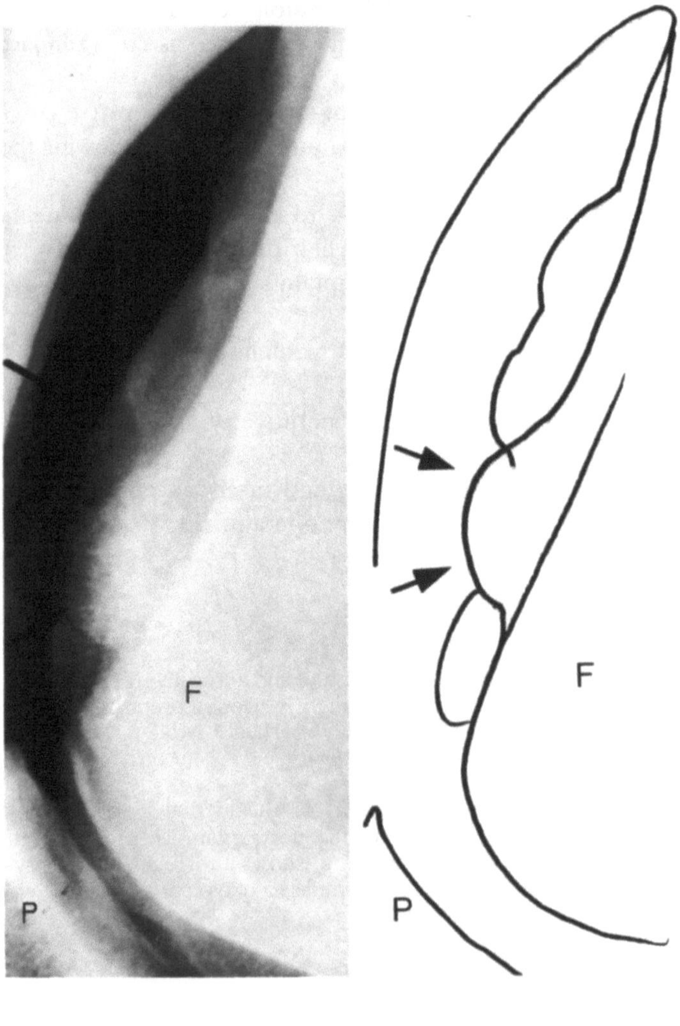

Fig. 4. Lateral view of the knee joint following air insufflation. Tumor *(arrow)* on the posterior wall of the suprapatellar pouch, directly above the patella. *P* = patella, *F* = femur

E. H., 34-year-old chauffeur:

Two months previously a sudden "giving-way" while running during soccer training. Since that time he could no longer forcefully extend his knee. Forced extension caused him great pain. Plain films showed no pathologic findings.

The arthrogram shows a protrusion half the size of a walnut in the floor of the suprapatellar pouch barely above the patella (Fig. 4).

Operation revealed a giant-cell tumor and confirmed the arthrographic findings. The patient's pain in full extension was produced by pressure of the patella against the tumor.

S. D., 31-year-old man:

Three months prior to examination the patient sustained a fall on the ice. Since then, increasing pain in the popliteal fossa and below the patella while walking and during knee flexion. Clinically the knee was unremarkable. No findings on plain film.

Arthrogram: Extraordinarily large villi extending into the joint from the infrapatellar fat pad (Fig. 5). Operation confirmed the finding: large fibrosed villi extending far into the joint (Hoffa's syndrome).

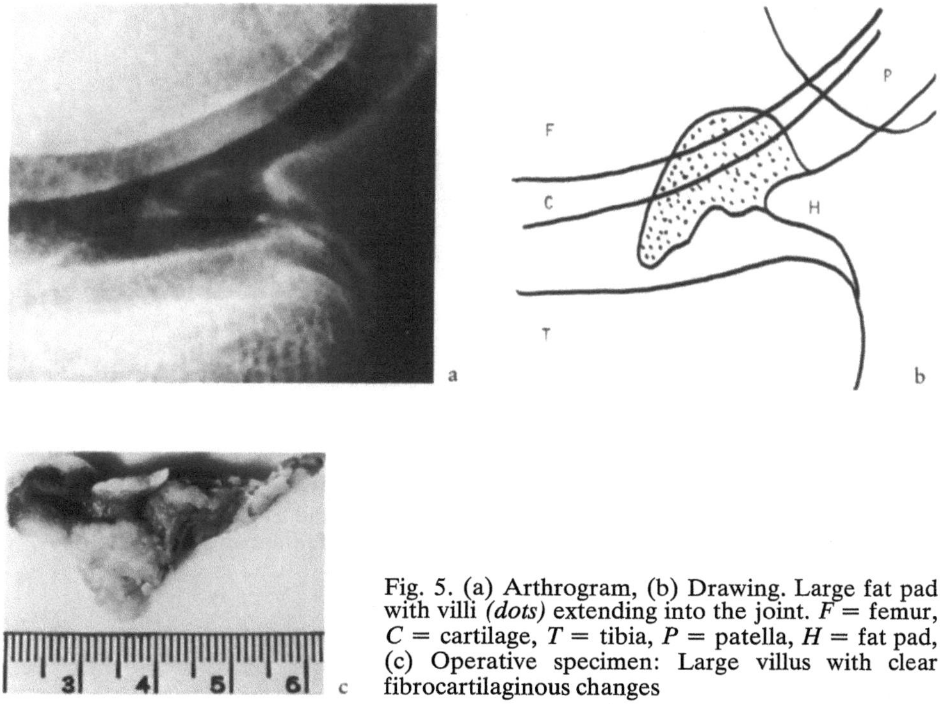

Fig. 5. (a) Arthrogram, (b) Drawing. Large fat pad with villi *(dots)* extending into the joint. F = femur, C = cartilage, T = tibia, P = patella, H = fat pad, (c) Operative specimen: Large villus with clear fibrocartilaginous changes

Meniscus Injuries

Clinically unequivocal meniscus injuries (Fig. 6) are no indication for arthrography unless there is some doubt as to the diagnosis, e. g., regarding lateral localization, etc.

M. M., 21-year-old housewife:

Patient presented with pain of several weeks' duration in the medial side of the knee joint, concentrated at the medial joint line. The pain was uncharacteristic; a snap could not be elicited. A medial meniscus lesion could not be excluded. No finding on conventional roentgenogram.

Arthrogram: Lateral discoid meniscus (Fig. 7).

Arthroscopy confirmed the finding.

Operation disclosed a large, almost totally discoid lateral meniscus.

Remarks: In this case arthrography gave a correct *lateral diagnosis* and prevented an operative intervention on the medial side.

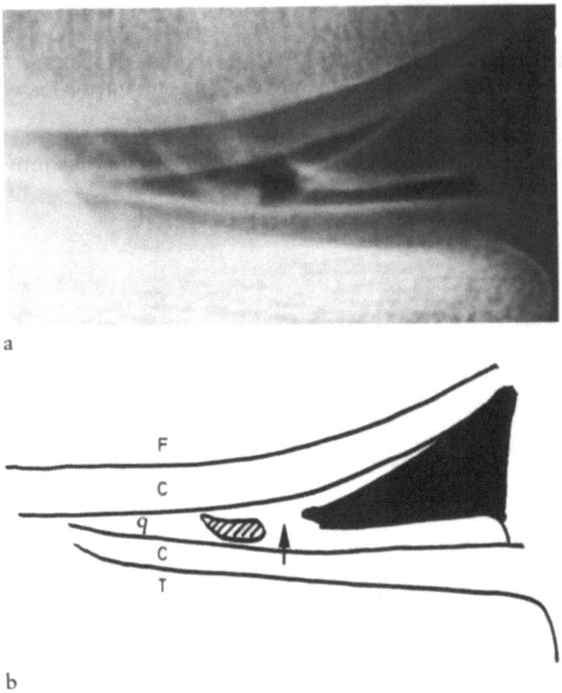

Fig. 6. Arthrogram of (a) a typical bucket-handle tear. Arrow in drawing indicates the site. *Black:* marginal remainder of the meniscus; *hatched:* the fragment, which forms the handle of the bucket. *F* = femur, *C* = cartilage coverings of femur and tibia, *T* = tibia

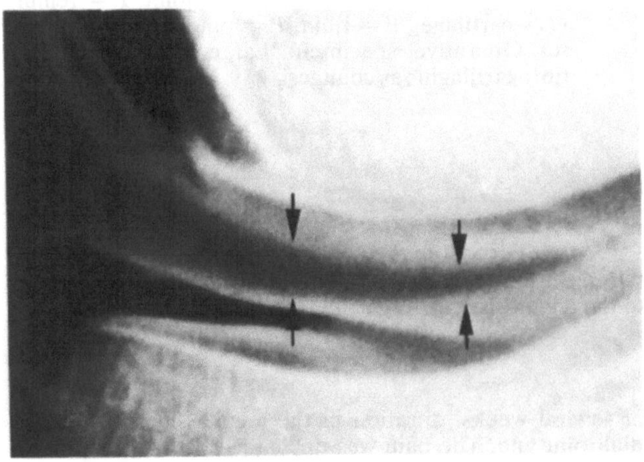

Fig. 7. Arthrogram of so-called discoid lateral meniscus reaching tongue-like deep into the joint *(arrows)*

K. M., 27-year-old man:

He had no recollection of any injury. A passionate mountain climber, he also works at a job which entails kneeling.

For several months, pain on weight bearing, increasing in the squatting position. No block to movement. The pain radiated to the lateral joint line. Meniscus lesion questionable.

Clinically the knee showed no signs of irritation. Pain on bending and rotating the foot to either side. Pain on pressure in the midpart of the lateral joint line.

Arthrography revealed a typical cystic degeneration of the lateral meniscus with a small horizontal tear (Fig. 8).

Confirmed at operation.

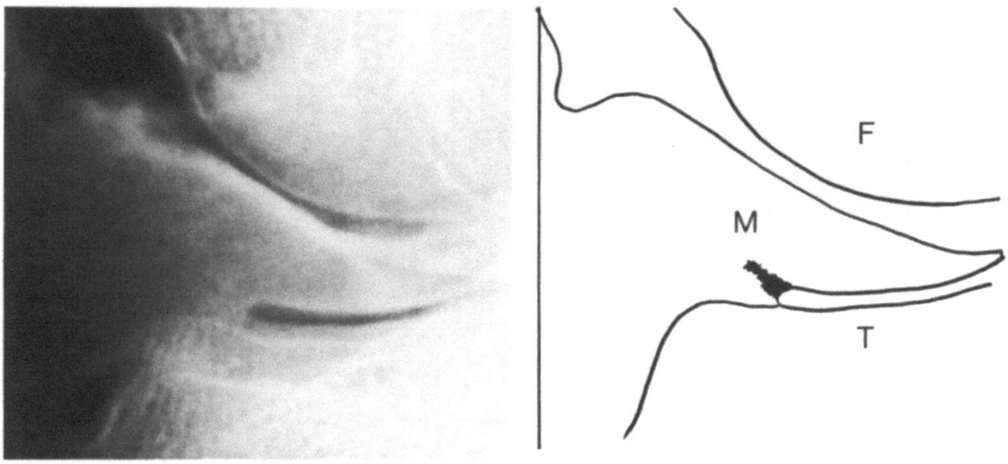

Fig. 8. Typical meniscus ganglion. The meniscus is crudely distended. A small horizontal tear at the undersurface in the area of the capsule is not clearly demonstrated here. See drawing. *M* = meniscus, *T* = tibia, *F* = femur

Post-Meniscectomy Status

B. C., 37-year-old civil servant:

At meniscectomy 3 years previous the mucoid degenerated and ruptured anterior portion of a meniscus was removed medially. At the time, arthrography was not done before operation due to the clear symptomatology. After resuming work, symptoms of something catching in the knee reappeared and increased in frequency. Initially, one suspected a lateral meniscus lesion.

Arthrography showed the avulsed remainder of the posterior horn of the medial meniscus (Fig. 9). Re-arthrotomy confirmed the finding. After removal the patient remains sympton-free.

Remarks: Arthrography furnished a clear indication for re-arthrotomy and also the exact localization of the finding (medial instead of lateral, as suspected clinically). A primary arthrography would probably have resulted in the usual subtotal meniscectomy in place of a partial resection.

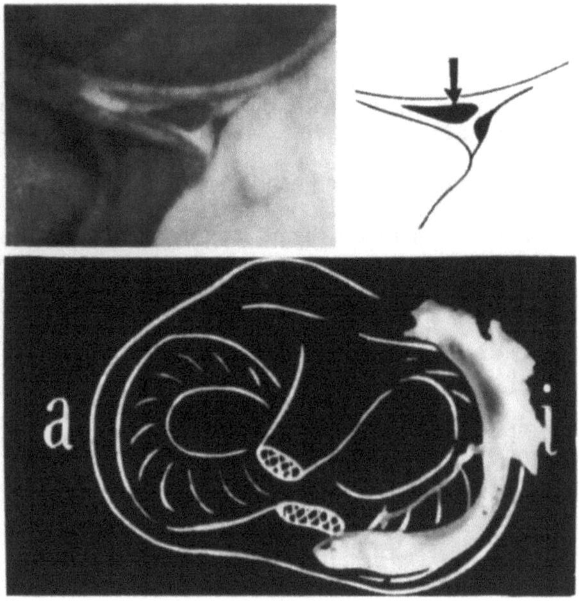

Fig. 9. *Above left:* Arthrogram; *right:* drawing; *below:* operative specimen. Post-meniscectomy arthrogram showing clearly a posterior horn fragment detached from the capsule *(arrow)*. Operative specimen shows the posterior horn fragment floating free in the joint

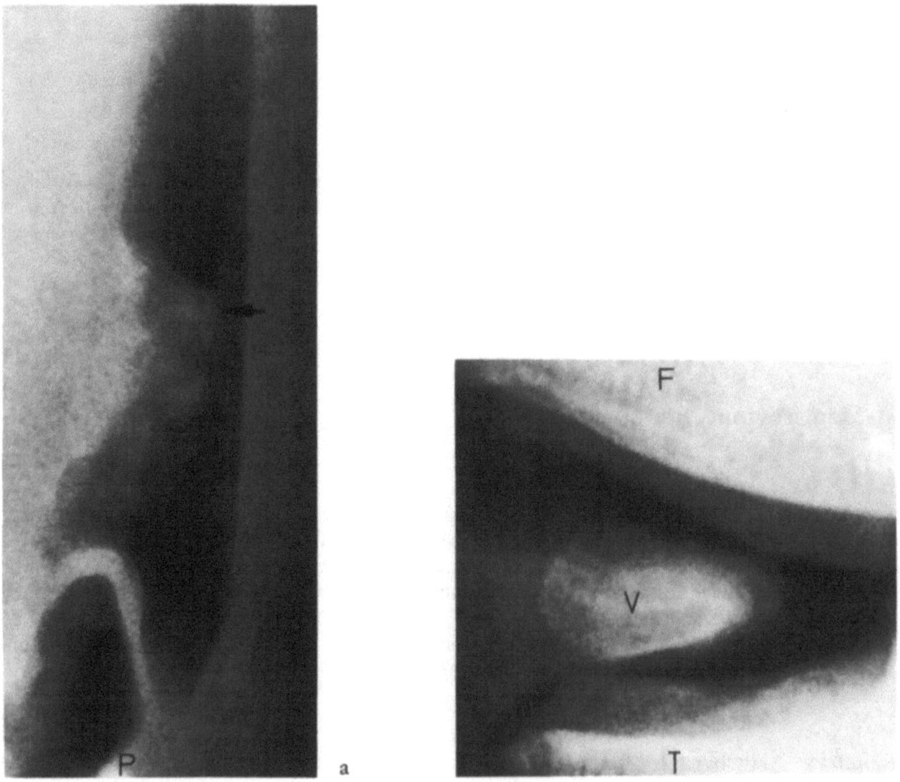

a b

Fig. 10. (a) Free-floating body in the suprapatellar pouch. *P* = patella at bottom of picture. (b) Ossification *(V)* of the meniscus. *F* = femur, *T* = tibia

Free-floating Interarticular Bodies and Chondromatosis

Free-floating interarticular bodies and detached chondromas may be found in any cavity of the joint. At times their localization can be determined only in part or not at all. In such cases arthrography makes a real contribution and helps in planning the operation (Figs. 10, 11).

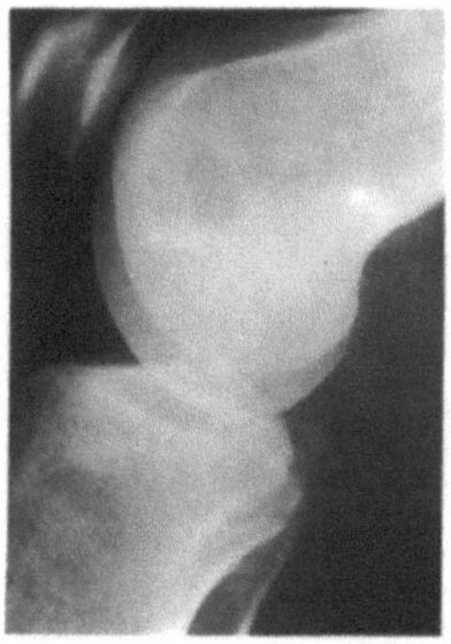

a

Fig. 11. (a) Plain film of the knee joint: pea-sized loose bodies above the border of the tibial head. (b) Arthrogram with drawing: The loose bodies *(black)* lie in the space between the torn medial meniscus *(striped,* posterior horn area) and the capsule

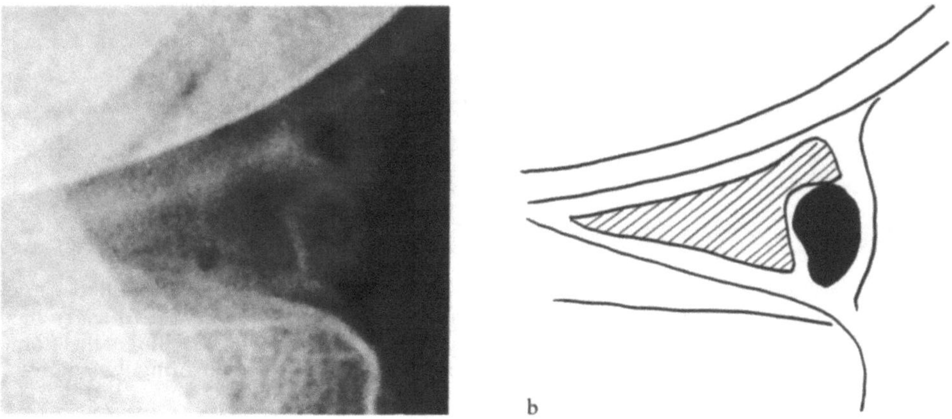

b

H. E., 36-year-old man:

In 1971 a lateral meniscectomy following a skiing accident. At the time of this operation cartilage damage was noted.

Since the operation the patient complained of lateral pains and feelings of loose bodies, also occasional giving way of the joint.

Plain film: Slight ossification in the lateral anterior articular space.

Arthrogram: Free-floating bodies in the suprapatellar pouch (Fig. 10a). The ossification in the anterolateral joint line lay within the stump of the meniscus (Fig. 10b).

Operation confirmed the diagnosis. The cartilaginous free-floating interarticular body in the superior pouch was removed and the ossified regenerated portion of the meniscus excised.

Osteochondritis Dissecans

The diagnosis can usually be made by plain films, but sometimes the question arises whether the joint mouse is already detached or whether, with an apparent detachment in the area of the bone, the *covering of articular cartilage* is still intact. Here arthrography plays a role regarding therapy and prognosis (Fig. 12).

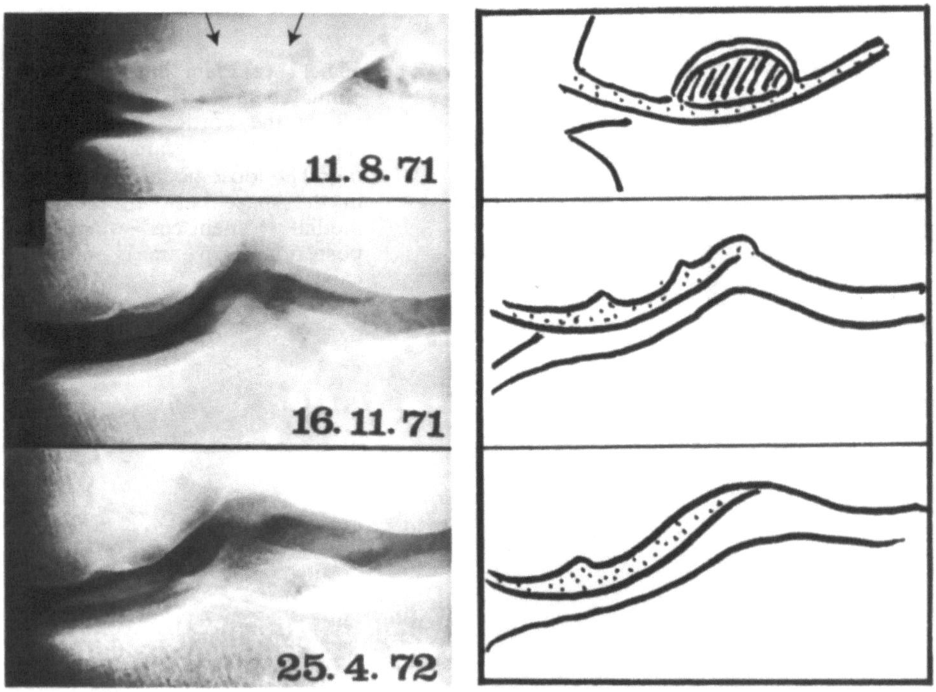

Fig. 12. Osteochondritis dissecans. Course of healing. Arthrogram: above, on 11-8-71, a distinctly intact cartilage covering in a clearly detached bony fragment. *Drawing:* the osseous fragment is cross-hatched, the cartilage stippled. On 16-11-71 the arthrogram shows partial consolidation of the bony fragment with the cartilage covering lying above it unchanged. The bony consolidation is more marked on 25-4-72

Chondropathy of the Patella

Chondropathy of the patella is in most cases a clinical diagnosis. Often roentgen studies for a long time reveal no unequivocal clues, neither plain films nor arthrograms. The posterior surface of the cartilage is hardly visible on arthrography. It can furnish, however, rough findings such as localized protrusions and swellings of the cartilage (Fig. 13) or a distinct thinning and destruction of the lamina (Fig. 14a, p. 109). Smaller alterations in cartilage are not demonstrable by today's arthrographic methods, but can be visualized very nicely by arthroscopy (Fig. 15b, p. 110).

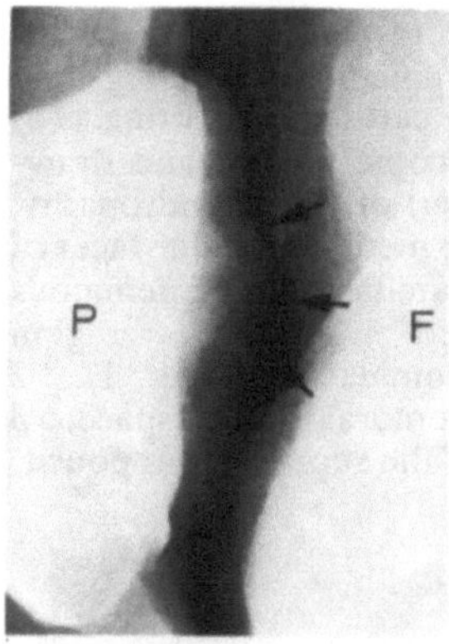

Fig. 13. Chondropáthy of the patella. Chondromalacia I. Localized swelling *(arrows)* of the patellar cartilage. *P* = patella, *F* = femur

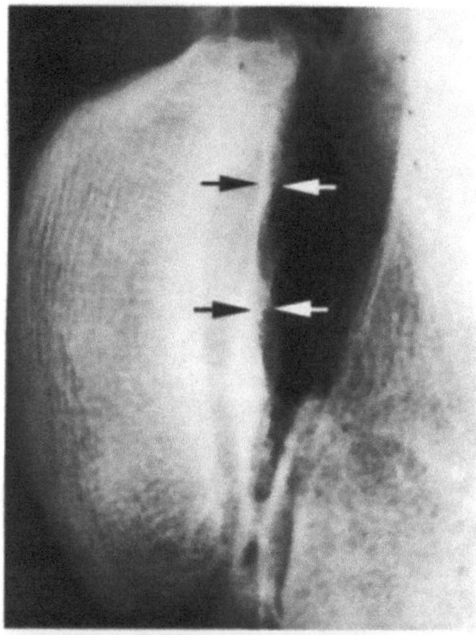
a

Fig. 14. (a) Lateral arthrogram of patella. Pronounced chondropathy: marked thinning and destruction of patellar cartilage *(arrows)*

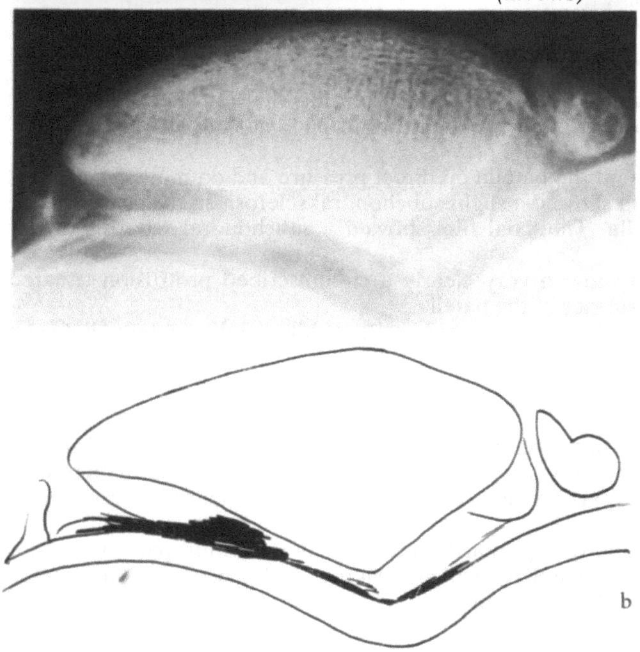
b

Fig. 14. (b) Axial arthrogram *(above)* and drawing *(below)*. Contrast medium imbibition *(black patches* in drawing) at destroyed patellar cartilage

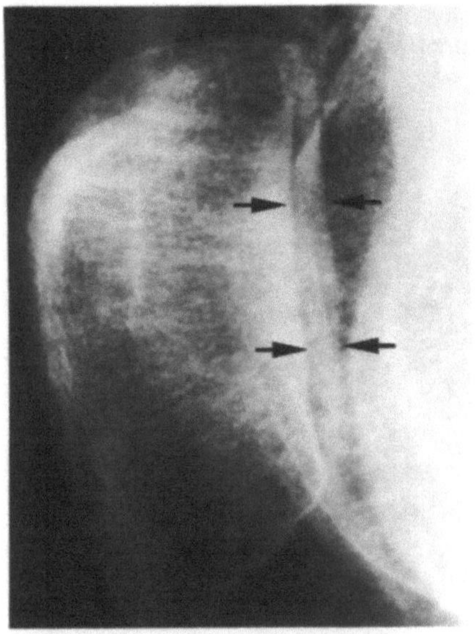

a

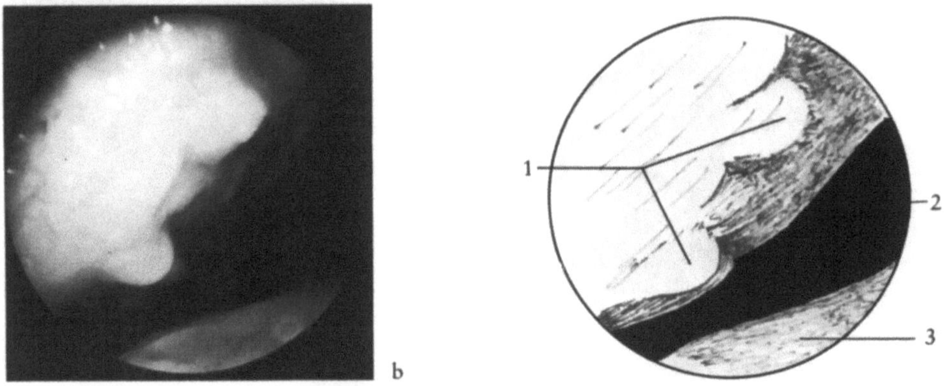

b

Fig. 15. (a) Patella with somewhat thinned but radiologically normal cartilage covering. (b) Arthroscopic picture and drawing *(right)* of this chondropathy, showing medial articular facet of the patella. *1* Edematous distended cartilage region (chondromalacia stage I). *2* Patellofemoral joint space. *3* Floor of the suprapatellar pouch

N. G., 30-year-old office worker:

One and one-half years previously, fell from a bicycle onto the left knee. Since then, intermittent discomfort of varying intensity behind both patellae, the left more severe than the right.

Clinically, distinct pain behind the patella on direct pressure and on movement under load. The plain roentgenogram showed a slight subchondral sclerosis in the center of the posterior surface of the patella. The axial film showed a subchondral sclerosis of the patella, decreasing laterally.

Air *arthrography* (Fig. 13) showed very clearly a circumscribed protrusion situated centrally on the cartilaginous surface of the patella.

At *operation,* a 1.5 cm malacic area was found in the middle patella centered between the facets.

H. A., 45-year-old housewife:

Fifteen years before, a fracture of the femur and fixation with a Küntscher nail. Removal of the Küntscher nail. Subsequently she received compensation because of persisting complaints in the right leg. Expert opinion: a psychogenic component and suspicion of hypochondriacal aggravation.

Plain roentgenogram: Osteoporosis, primarily in the area of the femoropatellar joint.

Arthrogram: Narrowing of the patellar cartilage together with a horizontal tear in the area of the posterior horn of the lateral meniscus.

Arthroscopy confirmed a pronounced chondropathy and the lesion of the lateral posterior horn (Fig. 15).

On the basis of the arthrogram the suspicion of a purely functional disorder had to be discarded.

Cartilage Lesions

In the future, arthrography may possibly prove to be useful in the supervision of arthroplasty of the knee. This applies particularly to those cases where the condition of the cartilage should be checked. Figures 16 and 17 show the status following meniscectomy due to a meniscus lesion and simultaneous screw-fixation of a detached fragment of cartilage. The postoperative cartilage condition may be easily evaluated.

P. A., 22-year-old soccer player:

Three years ago a meniscectomy of the lateral meniscus. Upon recommencing soccer play, a new injury and tear of the medial meniscus, which was also operated on.

The complaints persisted.

Arthrogram: Distinct tear of the cartilage.

A fragment of cartilage hung into the joint.

Operation confirmed the diagnosis. The cartilage was screwed on and healed completely.

The patient is again playing professional soccer.

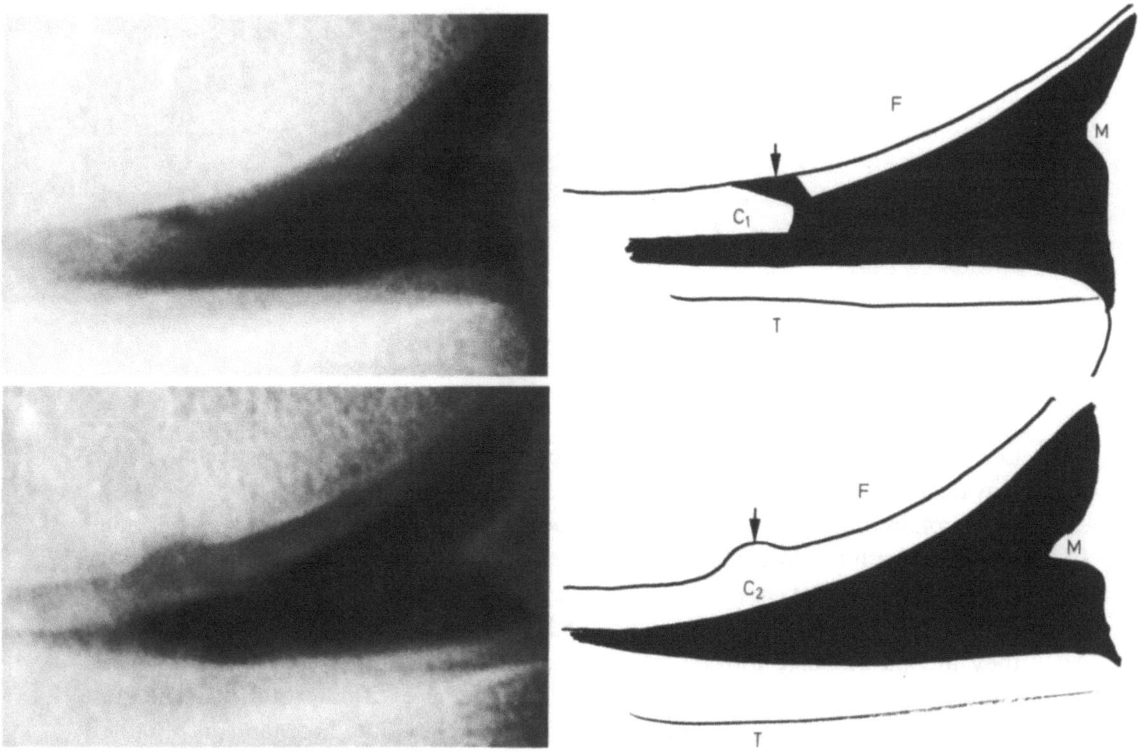

Fig. 16. *Above,* cartilage lesion *(arrow)*. C_1 = detached cartilage. *Below,* status after fixation and removal of screw (Dr. Raschle) *(arrow)*. C_2 = cartilage again growing in; M = meniscus regeneration following meniscectomy; F = femur; T = tibia

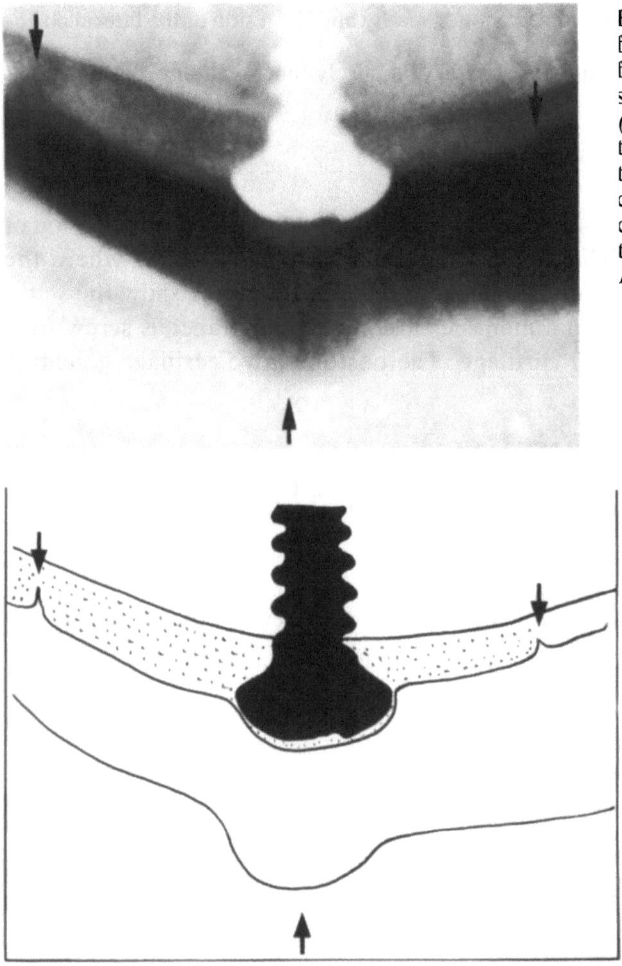

Fig. 17. Status after screw-fixation of a torn cartilage fragment, whose borders are still faintly recognizable *(arrows above)*. The head of the screw, itself covered by a thin, newly formed layer of cartilage, has produced a curved groove in the facing tibial cartilage *(arrow below)*. *Drawing:* cartilage dotted

Ligament Injuries

Lesions of the cruciate ligament occasionally go unrecognized, especially when they occur accompanying a lateral ligament or meniscus lesion.

The plain film of the knee joint may point to a cruciate ligament lesion if bone is torn off with the ligament at either the femoral or tibial attachment. However, such is not often the case.

In the arthrogram cruciate ligament lesions may usually be diagnosed when they are particularly looked for. The cruciate ligament is best shown on the lateral view with the knee in flexion and slight external rotation. The best demonstration, both of the anterior and posterior cruciate ligaments, is obtained when the joint is filled with air and then lateral tomograms are made in slight external rotation and flexion of the knee joint (van de Berg). Other views may be obtained depending on the initial findings.

Incomplete tears of the cruciate ligaments lead to irregularities in contour (Fig. 18), while complete tears reveal an evident narrowing of the cruciate

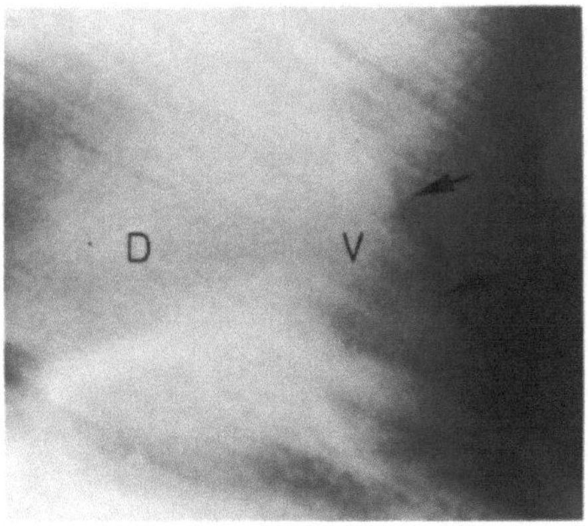

Fig. 18. Partial tear of the anterior cruciate ligament. Tomogram of cruciate ligaments in lateral projection. *V* = anterior cruciate ligament with concave anterior surface and nodular contours *(arrows)*. *D* = posterior cruciate ligament

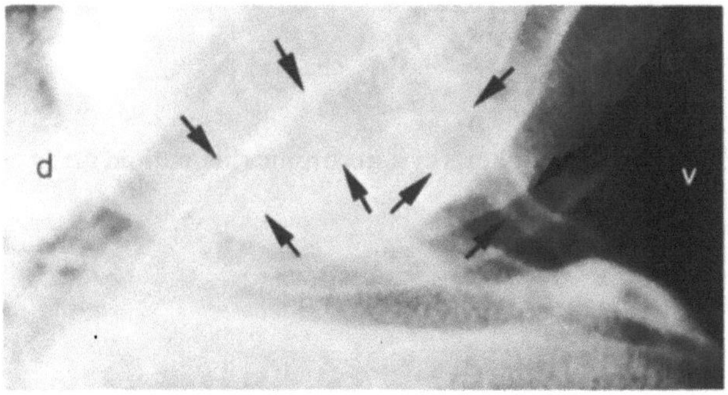

Fig. 19. Old lesion of the anterior cruciate ligament. Normal width of posterior cruciate ligament. Slight depression and thinning of the anterior cruciate ligament. *d* = posterior, *v* = anterior. Confirmed at operation (Dr. Raschle)

ligament shadow with concave anterior margins (Fig. 19). The operative finding then sometimes shows a synovial sheath in the case of older complete tears where the cruciate ligament itself is practically totally reabsorbed.

Injuries of the lateral ligaments and joint capsule are likewise demonstrable by arthrography through spot films or tomograms. However, in most cases the diagnosis is made clinically.

"Cysts" in the Popliteal Space

In the "irritated knee" of whatever pathogenesis, a frequent finding is a marked dilatation of the gastrocnemiosemimembranous bursa in the soft tissue of the popliteal space. This bursa is filled in flexion of the knee joint and is then very well visualized in the arthrogram. With the development of a complete closing off of this structure from the rest of the joint space, e.g., on an inflammatory basis, then a cyst is formed, the so-called Baker's cyst. This may also be demonstrated by posterior puncture and filling with contrast medium.

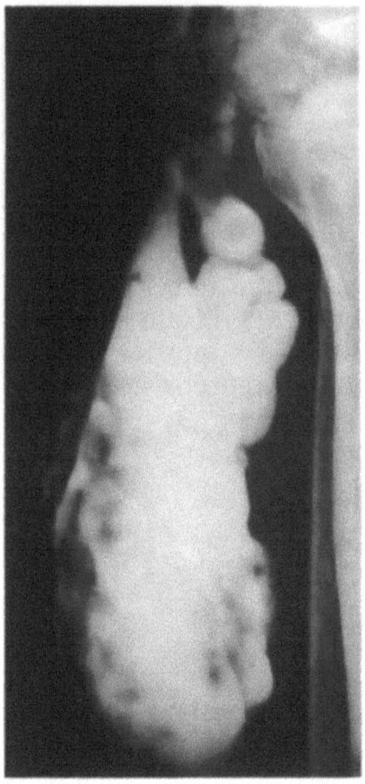

Fig. 20. Large Baker's cyst in chronic rheumatoid arthritis

Reliability of Arthrography

In general, according to our experience and the literature (see Fischedick), false diagnoses are made in 3–5% of cases. The result depends not so much on the choice of method as on the experience of the investigator, his technical precision and interpretation. Years of experience are necessary.

Summary

Contrast radiography of the knee joint is technically relatively simple and without complications. It provides an extensive view of the interior of the joint. Injuries and disorders of the meniscus, cartilaginous coverings, synovia, and capsule may be visualized. In many clinically doubtful cases it gives clear indications for further procedure, be it surgical or conservative treatment. The evidence provided by arthrographic findings depend, of course, upon the investigator, the technical performance and interpretation, but in general is extraordinarily reliable. In spite of this there are always cases in which even after a negative arthrogram and a long period of observation, the complaints and the suspicion of an internal lesion continue to exist. In such circumstances it may happen that despite negative arthrography an exploratory arthrotomy comes into question. Although arthrography markedly supplements the clinical findings, it does not replace them. The evaluation of a case is optimized when the trained physician, radiologist, and surgeon work together as a team.

References

Ahlbäck, S.: Acta radiol. (Stockh.) Suppl. **277** (1968)
Aufdermaur, M.: Schweiz. med. Wschr. **101,** 1405–1412, **39,** 1441–1445, **40** (1971)
Baumgartl, F., Dahm, A.: Zbl. Chir. **87,** 1916 (1962)
Candarjis, G.: La Médicale, No. spécial Noël, 17–20 (1955)
Catolla Cavalcanti, G., Cuzzupoli, F.: Minerva ortop. **20,** 105–118 (1969)
Croonenberghs, P., Rombouts, R.: J. belge Radiol. **36,** 481 (1953)
Del Buono, M., Rüttimann, A.: L'artrografia del ginocchio. Roma: Il Pensiero Scientifico Editore 1959
Ficat, P.: Arthrographie opaque du genou. Paris: Masson & Cie. 1957
Fischedick, O.: Z. Orthop. **106,** 759–765 (1969)
Fischedick, O.: Arthrographie des Kniegelenks. Handbuch med. Radiol. Bd. V/2. Berlin, Heidelberg, New York: Springer 1973
Geist, R. M., Whitsett, C. C., Hughes, C. R.: Brit. J. Radiol. **25,** 120 (1952)
Grösswang, F., Wruhs, O.: Endoscopy **2,** 164–168 (1970)
Jonasch, E.: Das Kniegelenk. Berlin: Walter de Gruyter & Co. 1964
Lindblom, K.: Acta radiol. (Stockh.) Suppl. **74** (1948)
Möhlmann, Th., Madlener, B.: Fortschr. Röntgenstr. **65,** 51–76 (1942)
Morscher, E.: Helv. chir. Acta **3,** 266 (1957)
Oberholzer, J.: Bruns' Beitr. klin. Chir. **158,** 113–156 (1933)
Reinhardt, K.: Radiologe **12,** 3, 77–86 (1972)
Ricklin, P., Rüttimann, A., Del Buono, M. S.: Die Meniscusläsion. Stuttgart: Georg Thieme 1964
Rieunau, G., Ficat, P., Rivière, R.: Acta orthop. belg. **20,** 421–445 (1954)
Rüttimann, A.: Röntgenfortschritte **87,** 736–755 (1957)
Rüttimann, A., Del Buono, M. S.: Chir. Praxis **1,** 107–120 (1959)
Schnauder, A.: Fortschr. Röntgenstr. **96,** 120–128 (1962)
Smillie, J. S.: Injures of the Knee Joint. Edinburgh: Livingstone 1946
Staple, T. W.: Radiology **102,** 311–319 (1972)
Van de Berg, A.: Encyclopédie Méd.-chir. (Paris) **1,** (1972)
Weston, W. J.: Brit. J. Radiol. **44,** 277–283 (1971)

English translation from the German edition *Der Orthopäde,* Vol. 3, pp. 166–177 (1974),

The Knee Joint of the Soccer Player (Its Stresses and Damages)

W. Müller*

Soccer, perhaps more than any other sport, places extraordinary demands on the function and capacity for resistance of the knee joint.

Apart from the externally induced injury that leads to such typical injuries as meniscus tears, osteocartilaginous shearing fractures and complex capsular-ligamentous injuries, the player's own bodily demands subject the knee to a maximum of stress in all directions.

Whereas injuries caused by direct impact with opponents are more common in other sports as, for example, American football, damage to the knee joint of the soccer player very frequently occurs spontaneously.

Therefore, we shall not discuss typical injuries such as meniscus lesions causing locking, capsular-ligamentous tears or dislocations of the patella. These lesions are well known in their own right and pose few problems for diagnosis and therapy. Also, these are injuries which usually occur as the result of an accident on the playing field caused by direct contact with an opponent. Instead, we shall go into the special conditions of stress and demand placed upon the knee of the soccer player, and in doing so describe many of the disorders that are encountered.

The chief reason for injury lies in the extreme rotatory demands on the knee joint in this sport. Fixation of the shoe in the ground by means of cleats in certain situations increases the peak stress which may end in self-induced trauma with tissue disruption of varying extent and the sequelae of hemarthrosis.

Therefore, for a symptom-free and fully efficient operational knee joint capable of meeting maximum stress in all imaginable situations, a controllable stability is a prerequisite.

The components which make for such stability lie partly in the inert structural features of the knee joint and in part in the elements that belong to the active element of the locomotor apparatus.

* Orthopädische Klinik (Director: Prof. Dr. E. Morscher), Chirurgisches Department der Universität Basel, Basel, Switzerland

Functional Considerations of Stability

The Pathophysiology of Inert Stability

Stability in extension is less of a problem, for in this case the rotatory movements are eliminated. The problem of stability becomes complex with the knee in increasing flexion because then not only must the angle of flexion be actively retained but also axial rotation must be controlled at specific angles, and, not least, lateral stability guaranteed in the varus and valgus directions.

In a normal functional sequence, undisturbed by secondary effects, a necessarily linked interdigitation of complex locomotor mechanisms is observed.

According to Dejour, in the supporting leg there are two positions at opposite extremes with full stability:

1. Flexion-valgus outward rotation
2. Flexion-varus inward rotation

Between these extremes there are many other functional positions in which a knee joint can be stable during the action of play. Figure 1 illustrates both positions in the same athlete. His left leg, still the supporting leg, is in flexion-varus internal rotation while the right leg, which will become the supporting leg immediately after kicking the ball, is in the opposite flexion-valgus external rotation.

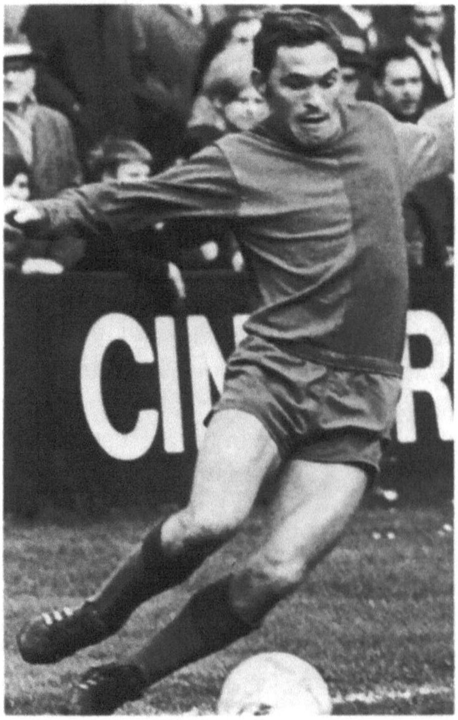

Fig. 1. Soccer player showing typical but stable extreme positions in regard to the knee joint. *Left leg:* flexion-varus internal rotation. *Right leg:* flexion-valgus external rotation (Photo Kurt Baumli, Basel)

Figure 2 shows the left supporting leg in flexion-valgus external rotation in the extreme stress of competitive action, while the kicking leg is in the opposing varus internal rotation position.

It follows from these descriptions that the crux of the problem of the knee joint in soccer is the question of maintaining stability in an infinite number of possible flexion rotation positions under maximum stress within the limits of the two opposing stable extreme positions.

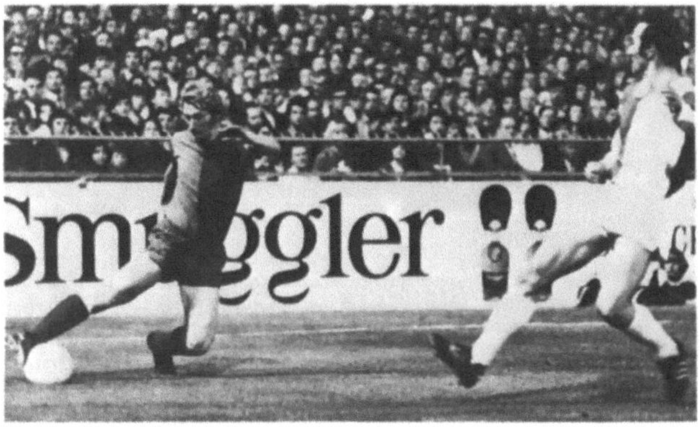

Fig. 2. Supporting leg of player *(left)* in stable extreme position. Flexion-valgus external rotation (Photo Kurt Baumli, Basel)

This stabilization places immense demands on all of the anatomical structures of the lower extremity.

It is completely out of date to think in terms of:
anterior cruciate ligament – anterior drawer
posterior cruciate ligament – posterior drawer
medial collateral ligament – medial stability
lateral collateral ligament – lateral stability

In opposing the above concept, the Americans Helfet, Hughston, Slocum, O'Donaghue and Nicholas, and to some extent their French followers Ficat, Trillat, Dejour and Bousquet have opened up new perspectives through their ideas and work. They have significantly enlarged the field of the pathophysiology of instability regarding aspects of rotation and posterior instability.

In the clinical interpretation of knee damage one can no longer think in terms of the above-mentioned ligaments. One speaks rather of the capsular ligamentous apparatus and considers its functional entirety in making judgments. In this connection, it is interesting to note that according to Casting et al., if the peripheral capsular ligamentous apparatus is left intact, a complete detachment of the anterior cruciate ligament produces an anterior drawer sign of only 2–3 mm! (The detachment is carried out through the longitudinal split cleft patellar ligament!) The anteromedial and to a lesser extent the anterolateral capsular elements are therefore in a position to further maintain anterior stability.

Here, one is also reminded of the good results obtained with the old external V-plasty replacement for the anterior cruciate ligament according to Smillie, in which the implant is drawn from the proximal attachment of the medial collateral ligament through the tibial tuberosity across to the proximal attachment of the lateral collateral ligament and there firmly sutured.

A further point is the importance of recognizing posterior stability or instability. Special consideration is given by the French authors to the so-called "coque condylienne" and by Hughston to the "posterior oblique ligament."

Posterior instability, similar to a cruciate ligament lesion, allows pathologic movements in the anteroposterior direction and especially when it occurs on only one side has a marked effect in the presence of the so-called rotatory instability (see Fig. 3).

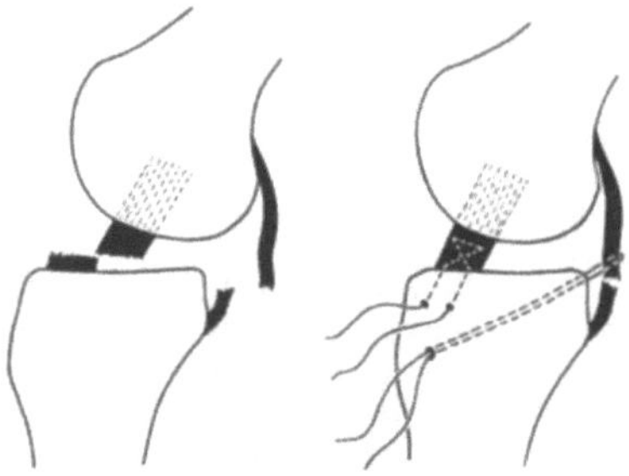

Fig. 3. Importance of posterior capsule instability compared with cruciate ligament instability in the anteroposterior direction

For example, if in a fresh medial ligament lesion the knee joint, in the fully extended position, can be opened out with valgus stress, then the posterior capsule must be torn. On the other hand, with the intact posterior capsule in full extension, it cannot be swung out laterally, even though, for example, the fibers of the medial collateral ligament may be completely detached. Then, if one flexes the knee 30 degrees, the posterior capsule relaxes and the medial capsular ligament instability can be appreciated (Fig. 4).

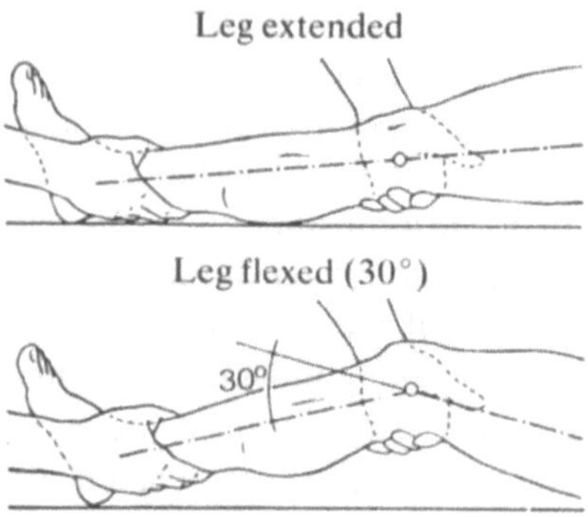

Fig. 4. Testing collateral ligament stability. In full extension an intact posterior capsule can simulate lateral stability. In flexion the posterior capsule relaxes and the collateral ligament instability becomes manifest

It is not within the scope of this paper to go into detail into the pathophysiology of knee joint instability or furnish a complete description of the subject. For this, the reader is referred to the pertinent literature (i.e., the works of the French and American authors cited above). In the paragraphs that follow, our special attention will be directed solely to the problem of rotatory instability.

Although Slocum (1968) and later Trillat, Dejour and Bousquet, and more recently Nicholas (1973) have called attention to this problem, this form of knee instability is still not widely appreciated. At the 1972 DGOT congress on ligament instability the subject went unmentioned by the official speakers. For that reason we reproduce Figure 5a–c which illustrates schematically the principle behind a rotatory instability and the method of examination according to Slocum.

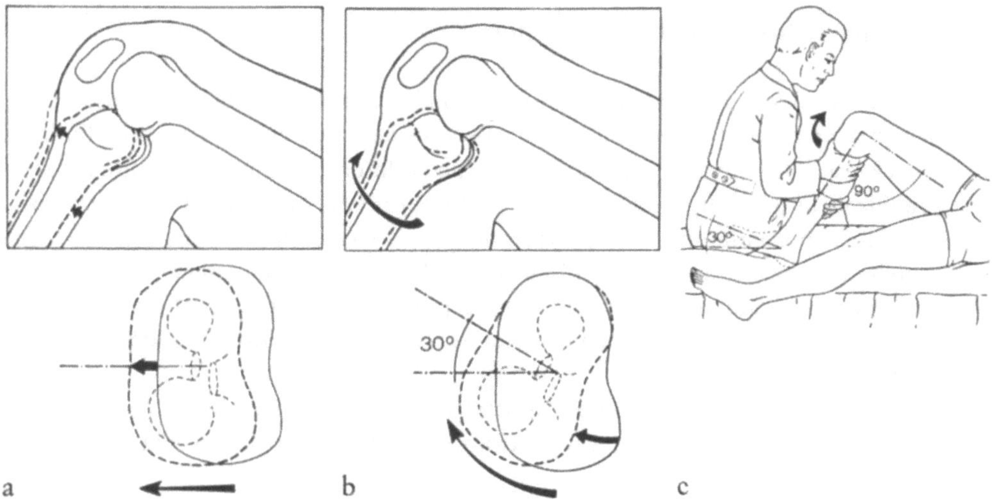

Fig. 5. (a) Normal anterior rotatory (drawer) instability. (b) Example of rotatory (drawer) instability. (c) Testing rotatory stability. In 60–90° flexion, by holding inward or outward rotation (the tip of the foot is held in place by the buttock of the examiner), the rotatory (drawer) stability is examined

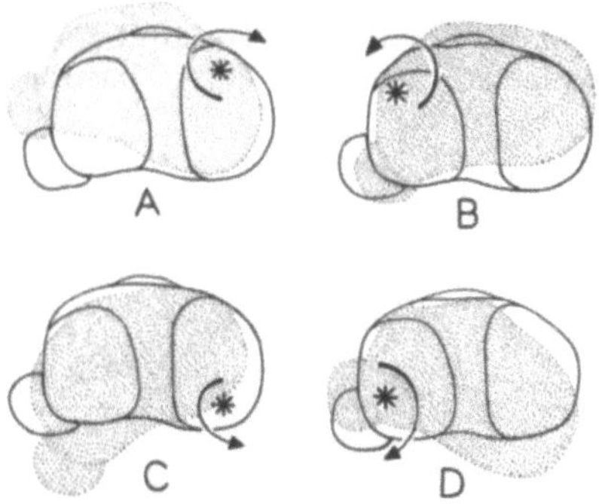

Fig. 6. Complex instabilities with displacement of the axis of rotation of the knee about the vertical axis: (a) anterolateral, (b) anteromedial, (c) posterolateral, (d) posteromedial

In his earliest work going back to 1973, Nicholas demonstrated four different rotatory instabilities, naming them, because of the multiple factors involved, complex instabilities. He classified them as anteromedial and anterolateral complex instabilities for the anterior region of the knee joint, and for the posterior region as posteromedial and posterolateral complex instabilities. The possible dislocations and changes in position of the articular pivot are shown in Figure 6.

Opposed to these are the simple instabilities such as loosening and the potential for abnormal movements about a single axis. On the other hand the complex instabilities are capable of displaying pathologic movements about several axes, for example lateral or medial instability in various positions of flexion, or with drawer and rotatory instabilitites. In fresh trauma complex instabilities are an absolute indication for operation to restore stability, whereas the simple instabilities may be treated conservatively.

Pathophysiology of Active Stabilization

In the extended position the powerful quadriceps muscle locks the knee joint while the capsule (coque condylienne) serves as a posterior buttress or limiting "backstop." On all sides, in addition to the collateral ligament apparatus, active stabilization medially to posteriouly and laterally, is provided by the sartorius, gracilis, semitendinous, semimembranous, gastrocnemius, biceps femoris, and popliteal muscles, and the iliotibial tract. Other passive auxiliary structures are the cruciate ligaments which, as rotating pillars of the knee joint, help to stabilize the axis of rotation, while both menisci follow the rotatory movements in the manner of movable brakes.

Out of these structures, one can form two correlating groups: "medial quadruple complex" and the "lateral quadruple complex" (Nicholas) (Fig. 7).

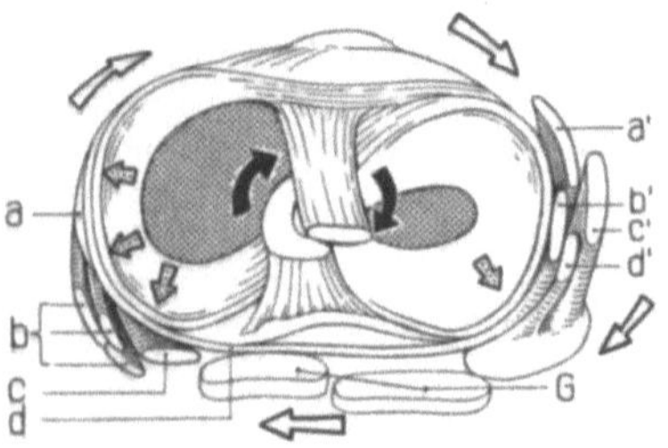

Fig. 7. The set of medial and lateral functional elements of the knee: medial and lateral quadruple complex with stress in valgus outward rotation. *a* Tibial collateral ligament, *b* Pesanserinus group (sartorius, gracilis and semitendinous,) *c* Semimenbranous. *d* Popliteal oblique ligament, *a'* Illiotibial tract. *b'*Popliteus. *c'* Biceps femoris. *d'* Fibular collateral ligament. *G* = Gastrocnemius

To the former belong:

a) The tibial collateral ligament
b) The pes anserinus with the tendons of the:
   - Sartorius muscle
   - Gracilis muscle
   - Semitendinous muscle
c) The semimembranous muscle
d) The posterior joint capsule with the "popliteal oblique ligament"

To the latter belong:

a) The iliotibial tract
b) The popliteal muscle
c) The biceps femoris
d) The fibular collateral ligament

These structures all have special importance for the stabilization of the knee joint. The popliteal muscle has the greatest effect on rotation, even in full extension. The considerable diameter of its tendon, which requires special care during surgery, explains the effective rotatory strength that the muscle imparts to the distal end of the femur.

Figure 8, another illustration of a soccer player in action, confirms the foregoing description.

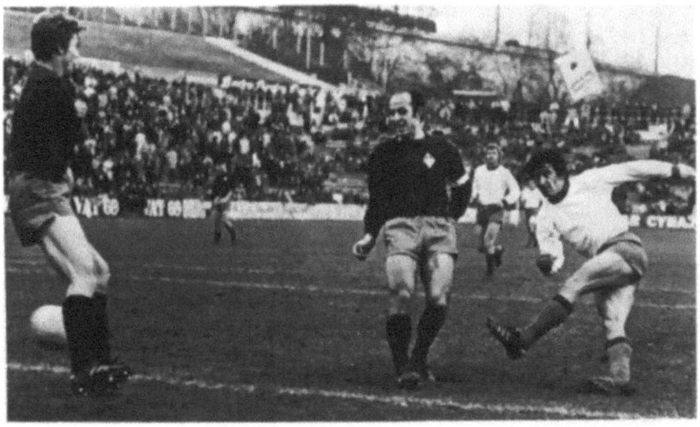

Fig. 8. A clear illustration *(right)* of full activity of the flexor-rotators even during the movement of extension. Right leg: muscles of the pes anserinus group (inward rotation). Left leg: iliotibial tract, biceps femoris (outward rotation) (Photo Kurt Baumli, Basel)

The player in the right of the figure is stabilizing both knee joints muscularly both with the extensors and the flexors while at the flexed knee the flexors primarily also act as rotators. In the right supporting leg, even in the extended position, one can observe the full contraction of the muscles belonging to the pes anserinus group (inward rotators). In the left leg, despite the vigorous extension resulting from just having kicked the ball, the laterally active components of outward rotation such as the iliotibial tract und the biceps femoris muscle are seen to be under full tension. With increasing tension the forces for rotation become greater (Fig. 9). This is of great importance inasmuch as the degree of effective possible rotation also increases.

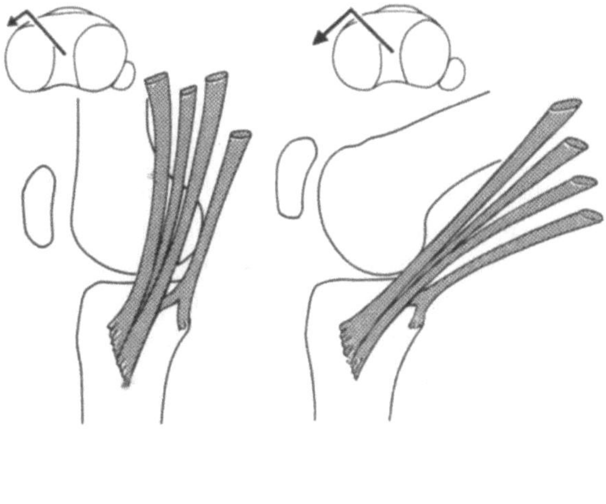

Fig. 9. Increase of rotation force of pes anserinus muscles with increase in angle of flexion

Rotation and Patellofemoral Components of the Knee Joint

Rotatory movements produce a shifting of the patella in relation to the femur. In acute peak demands this can lead to a dislocation. In all intermediate stages it leads only to an increased shearing effect on the cartilage. The vastus medialis with its direction of pull can, as the only extensor, counteract this lateralization (Fig. 10).

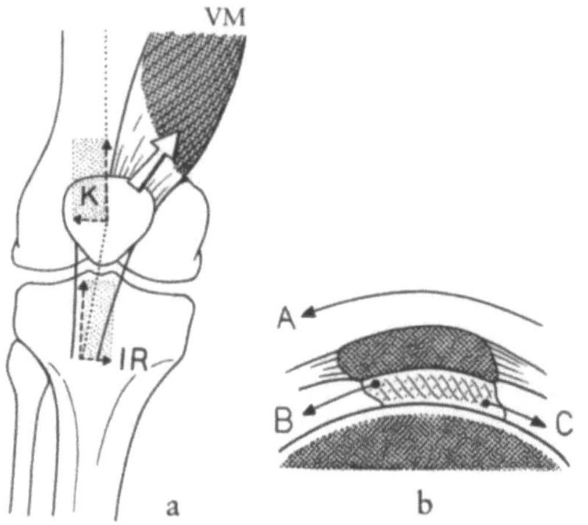

Fig. 10. (a) Effect of valgus components in quadriceps extension apparatus. *IR* Inward rotation of tibia. *K* Forces of patellar lateralization against the femur. *VM* Vastus medialis, which as the most important part of the extensors, must oppose lateralization of the patella. (b) Effect of patellar movement on more mobile superficial cartilage layer. *A* General direction of movement. *B* Same direction of deep cartilage covering. *C* Opposing direction of superficial cartilage covering

Thus, the vastus medialis has an exceedingly important function (Höhndorff, Ficat, Brenke and Weber). It must not be allowed to atrophy and in case of injury and especially after meniscus lesions it must be immediately exercised and trained. Should there be a loss of action due to atrophy, an as yet asymptomatic and latent chondropathy, as seen in fully compensated knee joints at operation, can become a painful annoyance. The deficit in the vastus medialis leads to new lateral shearing forces which can then act on the patellar cartilage (Fig. 10).

Not uncommonly this very fact results in a failure following meniscectomy, even though the meniscectomy, as for example in a bucket-handle tear, may be absolutely indicated.

Rotatory Movement and the Menisci

During rotation, both menisci participate in considerable shifting on the tibial plateau (Fig. 11). According to Lanz-Wachsmuth, this leads to a quite special type of stress, less so in knees with active well-controlled and stable rotation than in loose knees. Obvious meniscus tears represent little difficulty in diagnosis. Much more difficult is the evaluation in subtle meniscus lesions. Loose knees are injured more frequently in their ligamentous area (Nicholas, 1970). According to Ficat (1962), Trillat (1971) and Höhndorff (1972), there is a connection between laxity and meniscus pathology. In all probability, loosening of the posterior horn and formation of meniscus tears are quite common. Many bucket-handle tears in "true" meniscus trauma orginate in a preexisting tear of the posterior horn. Often the result is not a clear bucket-handle formation but rather a degenerative form of meniscus lesion. Ficat speaks of a "meniscosis" and Höhndorff of "meniscopathies."

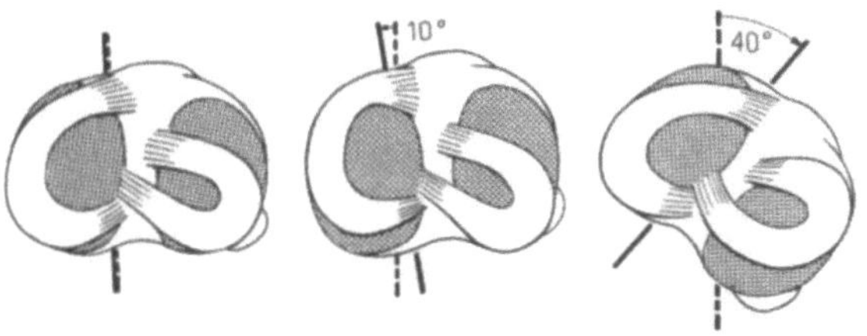

Fig. 11. Shifting of meniscus on tibial plateau in flexion, internal and external rotation

This type of knee also shows a tendency to further complaints following meniscectomy, because by itself it produces too great a rotatory laxity. Should a meniscus be removed from such a knee the excessive rotatory demands placed on the remaining meniscus will cause immediate pain since every meniscectomy, at least temporarily, bequeaths an increased rotatory instability. If this does not improve spontaneously and if rotatory instability and complaints persist for months following meniscectomy, then an operation such as Slocum's "pes-anserinus transplantation" should not be delayed because instability encourages, in addition, development of arthroses (Bühler, 1973; Debeyre and Artigon, 1973).

In his discussion of "meniscopathies" Höhndorff speaks of biological inferiority predisposing a knee to derangement. The course of this process is accelerated through its special function. According to the results of his follow-up of 113 soccer players with meniscectomies, of which 56 were designated good to very good, and 20 as bad, in the latter group we find such "meniscopathies" to be particularly numerous. Fifteen of them were only operated on months after the event (accident) leading to decompensation. This demonstrates how difficult the diagnosis and indications for surgery often are in these patients. It is certain that false diagnoses are more common in such cases than in patients with a clear and unambiguous meniscus block.

In 1930 Finochietto coined the term "signo del salto" to describe the ascent of the femoral condyle onto the posterior horn. This clicking sound is often describ-

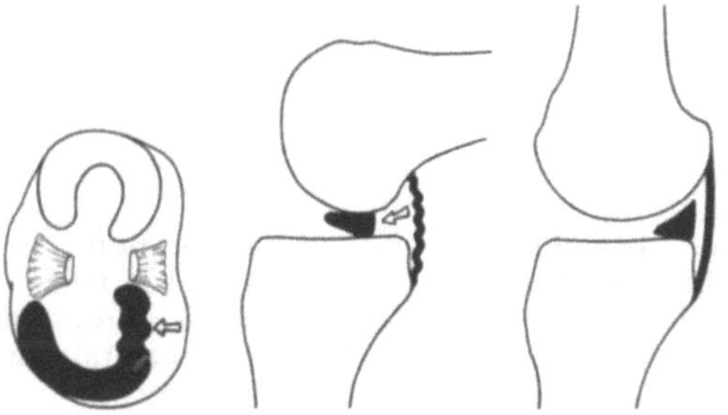

Fig. 12. Femoral condyle ascending onto loose posterior horn of the meniscus. Finochietto's "signo del salto"

ed by patients as a sort of giving way during which the knee suddenly feels unstable (Fig. 12).

Hence, it is understandable that Trillat compiled his classification of meniscus tears according to tears of the posterior horn (Fig. 13).

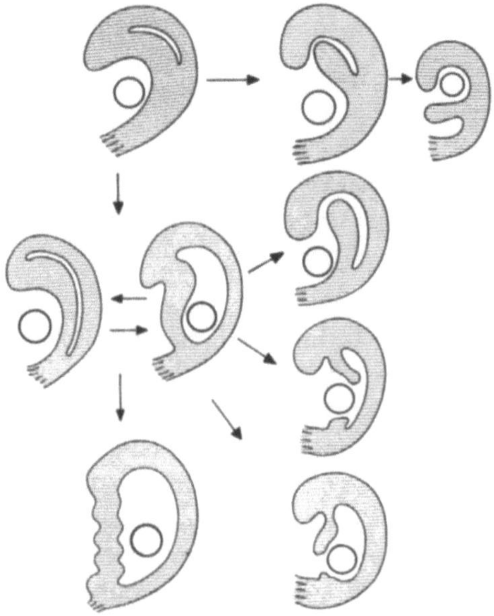

Fig. 13. Pathogenetic classification of various meniscus tears according to posterior horn tears (stage I) (Trillat) O = position of condyle

Rare Disturbances Caused by Extreme Rotatory Stress

a) Dislocations and Partial Dislocations of the Fibular Condyle

With a flexion of the knee joint of about 90 degrees, the biceps femoris muscle draws the head of the fibula posteriorly. In a loose tibiofibular joint this results in an isolated rotation of the fibular condyle about its long axis where the lateral collateral ligament forms the axis of rotation.

This syndrome, occasionally observed by us in cases of isolated pain in the lateral region of the knee joint, can lead to complete dislocation. Up to now, we

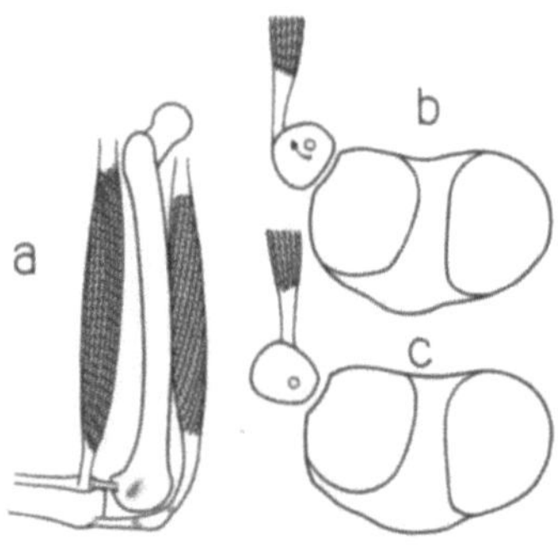

Fig. 14. Fibular condyle dislocation. (a) Schematic diagram of biceps traction in flexion. (b) Rotary action of biceps with axis of rotation about point of insertion of fibular collateral ligament. (c) Resulting rotation dislocation

have observed six such cases. Reposition can follow spontaneously by manipulation while rotating the knee or by digital compression after i.v. administration of a relaxant such as Valium (Fig. 14).

b) Fibular Nerve Compression Syndrome

As a result of the special stress in the area of the proximal fibula and the considerable traction of the fibular muscles, the passage for the fibular nerve at the neck of the fibula can become narrowed. Lateral lower leg pain occurring with activity can be the result. The EMG shows innervation disturbances and the conduction velocity is diminished. Similarly to carpal tunnel release, release of the canal results in a cure of symptoms.

c) Infrapatellar and Saphenous Compression Syndrome

This nerve can likewise be constricted at its point of exit from the fascia. Also, it may cause pain following contusions and in both cases mimic a symptomatology with pain on rotation medially in the area of the joint line. This fact must always be taken into consideration in the differential diagnosis. Infiltration of the area with a local anesthesia helps to clarify the matter and secure the diagnosis of an extra-articular disturbance. Treatment consists of releasing the restraining fascia (Meier, 1970).

d) Tendon Insertion Complaints

Besides the disturbances described above, one finds in soccer, as in other sports, disorders of tendons and ligaments at their points of bony attachment. The point of insertion of the fibular collateral ligament into the fibular condyle is a particularly frequent example. Exact knowledge of the anatomy and function will clarify the relationship. According to Suckert (1950) tendon disorders are as a rule more frequent in juveniles.

Discussion

The knee joint of the soccer player can exhibit all the disturbances that are possible in a knee joint. Very common are meniscus lesions (Winkelmann, Höhndorff, Basch, Denner, Ehricht, Idelberger, Knoll, Plattner, Weber, Zippel, Zoss), but the examining physician must not be misled into initially suspecting a meniscus lesion in every case. On the contrary, on account of the possibility of a false diagnosis, other lesions must first be excluded. A complete and detailed clinical examination and evaluation of the history is indispensable. Essentially weak knee joints clearly present more problems. In addition to the osteochondral disturbances, which are discussed by Wagner elsewhere in this volume, the main attention should be focused on the problem of stability about every possible axis of movement in the knee joint. In soccer, rotatory stability plays a leading role. Figure 15 illustrates the forces and dynamics of the functional demands of the knee joint. The correct explanation for the various conditions can thus be more easily understood.

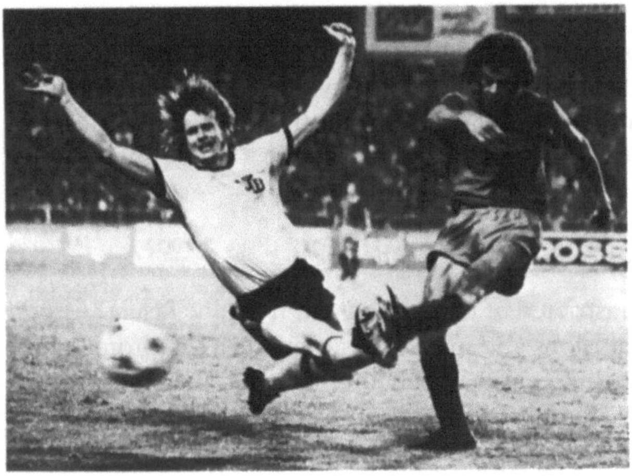

Fig. 15. Forces and dynamics of functional stress on knee joint (Photo R. Grossenbacher, Basel)

Summary

The knee joint of the soccer player is subject to extreme stress of a very special nature. Only a knee joint that is actively and passively stable in every respect can be safely put into action. The importance of rotatory stability is clarified by putting it in this pathophysiologic context.

References

Bandi, W.: Helv. chir. Acta Suppl. **11,** (1972)
Brenke, H., Weber, J.: Ther. Prax. Körperkult. **21,** 152 (1972)
Bühler, A.: Gonarthrose und Tibiaosteotomie. Dissertation. Basel 1973
Burri, C., Hutschenreuter, P., Radde, J.: Exerpta med. **298,** 4 (1973)
Castaing, J., Burdin, Ph., Mougin, M.: Rev. Chir. Orthop. **58,** Suppl. (1972)
Dettlof, M.: Med. Sport. **44,** 225 (1970)
Debeyre, J., Artigou, J. M.: Rev. Chir. Orthop. **59,** 641 (1973)
Dreisilker, U.: Gefahren der lokalen Corticosteroid-Injektion an der Achillessehne. 24. Sportärztekongreß Würzburg, 14.–17. Oktober 1971
Ficat, P.: Pathologie fémoro-patellaire. Paris: Masson 1970
Ficat, P.: Pathologie des ménisques et des ligaments du genou. Paris: Masson 1962
Finochietto: El signo del Salto (cited in Ficat. P.) Press. Med. Argentina. Juni (1930)
Goodfellow, J. W., Hungerford, D., Woods, D. C., Zindel, M.: J. Bone Jt Surg. B **56,** 198 (1974)

Heiss, F.: Praktische Sportmedizin. Sportärztliche Untersuchungen und Beratungen. Stuttgart: Enke 1974
Helfet, A. J.: The Management of Internal Derangement of the Knee. Philadelphia: J. B. Lippincott 1963
Henche, H. R.: Z. Orthop. **111,** 523 (1973)
Höhndorf: Med. Sport **12,** Heft 3 (1972)
Houghston, J. C.: J. Bone Jt Surg. **A 50,** 1003 (1968)
Houghston, J. C., Eilers, A. F.: J. Bone Jt Surg. **A 55,** 923 (1973)
Houghston, J. C., Stone, M., Andrews, J. R.: J. Bone Jt Surg. **A 55,** 1318 (1973)
Jani, L., Müller, W., Dolanc, B.: Ther. Umsch. **30,** 260 (1972)
Kopell, H. P., Thompson, W. A. L.: Peripheral Entrapment Neuropathies. Baltimore: Williams and Wilkins 1963
Maquet, P., Simonet, J., De Marchin, P.: Rev. Chir. Orthop. **53,** 11 (1967)
Mauk, H. P.: J. Bone Jt Surg **A 18,** 984 (1936)
Meier, W.: Z. Unfallmed. Berufskr. **63,** 129 (1970)
Morscher, E.: Reconstr. Surg. Traumat. **12,** 2 (1971)
Morscher, E.: Orthop. Praxis **6,** 31 (1970)
Morscher, E., Müller, W.: Therap. Umschau, **31,** 227 (1974)
Morscher, E., Pfeiffer, K. M.: Z. Unfallmed. Berufskr. **1,** 47 (1970)
Nicholas, J. A., Freiberger, R. H., Killoran, P. J.: J. Amer. med. Ass. **212,** 2236 (1970)
Nicholas, J. A.: J. Bone Jt Surg. **A 55,** 899 (1973)
O'Donoghue, D. H.: J. Bone Jt Surg. **A 32,** 721 (1950)
O'Donoghue, D. H.: J. Bone Jt Surg. **A 48,** 503 (1966)
O'Donoghue, D. H.: J. Bone Jt Surg. **A 55,** 941 (1973)
Ogden, J. A., Southwick, W. O.: J. Bone Jt Surg. **A 55,** 1319 (1973)
Outerbridge, R. E.: J. Bone Jt Surg. **B 46,** 179 (1964)
Owen, R.: J. Bone Jt Surg. **B 50,** 342 (1968)
Pipkin, G.: Clin. Orthop. **74,** 161 (1971)
Pipkin, G.: J. Bone Jt Surg. **A 32,** 363 (1950)
Plsek, J.: Chirurgisches Vademecum des Sportarztes. München-Gräfeling: Werk-Verlag Dr. Edmund Nanaschewski
Ricklin, P., Rüttimann, A., Del Buono, M. S.: Meniscus Lesions. Practical Problems of Clinical Diagnosis, Arthrography and Therapy. New York and London: Grune + Stratton, 1971
Roberts, E. M., Metcalf, A.: Mechanical analysis of kicking. Medicine and sport: Biomechanics I, 1st. Int. Seminar Zürich (1967) (ed.) Jokl, E. Basel, New York 1968
Slocum, D. B., Larsen, R. L.: J. Bone Jt Surg. **A-50,** 226 (1968)
Slocum, D. B.: J. Bone Jt Surg. **A 50,** 211 (1968)
Smilie: Injuries of the Knee Joint. Edinburgh: Livingstone 1946
Suckert, R.: Tendopathie am Kniegelenk und ihre Behandlung. Österreich, J. Sportmedizin **1,** 24 (1971)
Trillat, A., Dejour, H., Couette, A.: Rev. Chir. Orthop. **50,** 813 (1964)
Trillat, A., Dejour, H.: Rev. Chir. Orthop. **53,** 331 (1967)
Trillat, A., Dejour, H., Bousquet, G.: Lyon: Simep éditions (1971)
Trillat, A., Ficat, P.: Rev. Chir. Orthop. **58,** Suppl. I 32 (1972)
Winkelmann, B.: Meniscusschaden beim Sportler. 24. Sportärztekongreß in Würzburg, 14.–17. Oktober 1971
Zippel, H.: Meniscusverletzungen und Meniscusschäden. Leipzig: Johann Ambrosius Barth 1973

English translation from the German edition *Der Orthopäde,* Vol. 3, pp. 193–200 (1974),

Trauma-Induced Chondromalacia Patellae

W. Bandi*

The etiology of chondromalacia patellae is very complex and, in specific cases, cannot always be clearly delineated. The macroscopic picture of the malacic cartilage indicates *mechanically* damaged tissue. A histological examination, however, reveals degenerative changes of the cartilage which in turn question the mechanical etiology. Its clinical course presents additional obstacles to the pathogenetic explanation: at times complaints start immediately after an accident, at other times only after a certain latent period. It is also noteworthy that chondromalacic damages with an entirely latent clinical course are frequently found incidentally in connection with arthrotomies performed for various indications or even at post mortem examination [1, 20, 21].

This paper examines the possibility of chondromalacia patellae resulting from an isolated trauma such as an accident. This question is of considerable importance since, as a forerunner of femoropatellar arthrosis [1, 3, 5, 12, 16, 25], chondromalacia patellae can determine the future of a knee joint.

Several authors have described the pathogenesis of chondromalacia patellae. The presumption of important endogenous factors of the joint mechanism or of trophic factors [9, 13, 22, 23] stands in the way of a total acceptance of the theory of traumatic origin [1, 6, 10, 16, 18]. Since neither the clinical course nor the pathologicoanatomic picture permit an etiological evaluation of accident-caused isolated injuries, this question shall be dealt with here on the basis of the functional structure of the cartilage.

The Functional Structure of Hyaline Articular Cartilage

According to Benninghoff's investigations [4] hyaline articular cartilage represents a compound system consisting of three elements: *chondrocytes* and *collagen fibrils,* both embedded in a hyaline *ground substance* in accordance with a certain pattern. This compound system is capable of repeatedly enduring powerful pressures within physiological limits without suffering any damages or lasting deformities. A vertical section through the hyaline articular cartilage shows four different zones:

* Surgical Department, Bezirksspital (Chief: Dr. med. Bandi), Interlaken, Switzerland

First, a shiny and smooth *tangential zone* which forms the articular surface; below that a narrow *transitional zone,* then a *perpendicular* or *pressure zone* which constitutes more than half of the thickness of the joint and finally a narrow *calcified zone* where the articular cartilage adheres to the subchondral bone. The character of the individual zones is determined by the orientation of the collagen fibrils.

Anchored in the calcified zone, these fibres rise vertically through the *perpendicular* or *pressure zone* and cross one another approximately between the third and the fourth quarters close to the surface (transitional zone). Finally they run in a flat, increasingly elongated arc tangentially towards the border of the cartilage where they flow into the synovial coat and into the periosteum. On the articular surface itself, i.e. removed from the border of the cartilage, the collagen fibrils form an arc in the tangential zone, then return vertically into the perpendicular zone and finally reattach in the calcified zone. They thus form a bow whose vertical sides are subject to an increasing tension when under strain (see below). The course of these fibres determines also the orientation of the individual chondrocytes which are either globular or grouped in round nests. The entire system is filled out and functionally integrated by the hyaline ground substance.

Benninghoff has demonstrated that in their course the collagen fibrils envelop the globular chondrocyte formations in a *circular web.* The functional units thus created are called chondrones. Different chondrones, being in their turn enveloped, form larger or smaller bundles. This structure determines the specific function of the hyaline articular cartilage. The spherical body, in this case represented by chondrocytes, or chondrocyte agglomerates, comprises the greatest content with the smallest surface. Every deformation of the sphere entails an increase of its surface. Therefore every deformation stretches the collagen fibrils in the chondrone. Since the fibrils are anchored in the calcification zone as well as in the periosteum, any pressure causes increased tension in the cartilage and thus a force which counteracts the deformation. This means that forces acting upon the cartilage, within physiological limits, result in an increase of the modulus of elasticity within the cartilage. This mechanism, which Benninghoff had postulated in theory, was confirmed (Fig. 1) through the experiments of Hirsch [13].

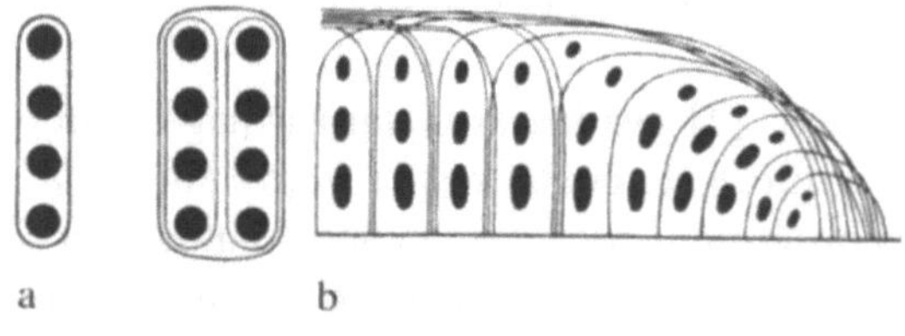

Fig. 1. Hyaline articular cartilage in schematic representing the compound structure. (a) Each circular disc represents a chondrone as a functional unit: a chondrocyte enveloped circularly and in several layers by collagen fibrils (not shown here). On the left four and on the right eight chondrones are united in a bundle. (b) General course of the fibrils inside the hyaline articular cartilage. For reasons of clarity the individual wrapping of the chondrone bundles *(black ovals)* has been omitted (after A. Benninghoff)

This mechanical situation together with the content of glycosaminoglycans in the hyaline intercellular substance determine jointly the elasticity of the cartilage [13, 22, 28]. A pathologic reduction of the elasticity is usually accompanied by a decrease in glycosaminoglycans in the perpendicular zone.

Not only is this functional microanatomical organization important for the articular mechanism in that friction is recuced, but it also plays a vital part in the nutrition of the cartilage. The articular cartilage, being an avascular tissue, depends for its nutrition on diffusion, mostly on nutrients from the synovial fluid [8, 14]. The pressures caused by the movement of the joint create a thorough kneading of the cartilage. Through alternating pressure and suction they activate the diffusion to a degree which is proportional to the extent of the elastic deformation (similar to the lifting of a pump).

Any loss of elasticity of the hyaline articular cartilage exposes it to greater wear as a result of increased friction and simultaneously impairs its nutrition (Fig. 2).

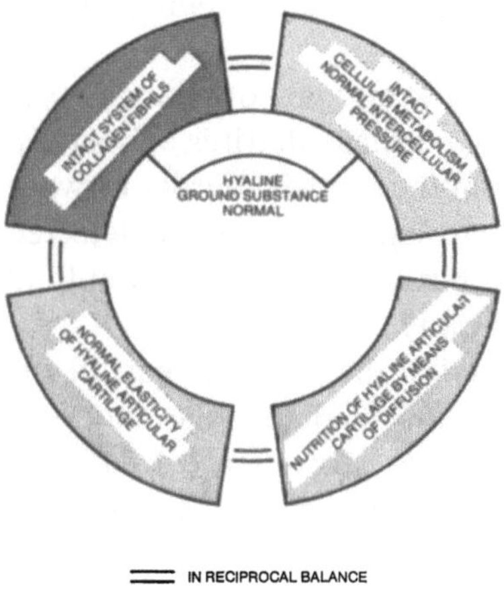

Fig. 2. Representation of interdependence of structure and function of hyaline articular cartilage

Pathological Anatomic Aspects

Chondromalacia patellae arises from wear of various etiology and presents three grades of severity [10].

Grade 1: In a circumscribed area the articular cartilage shows a loss of brightness together with a yellowish or brownish-grey discoloration. This area appears to be slightly elevated in comparison with the healthy cartilage and, upon palpation with a probe, shows a diminished elasticity.

Grade 2: Fissuring or separation of the cartilage into fascicles in a circumscribed area. The fissures run vertically or diagonally to the surface. Individual fascicles can become swollen, villus-like. The fissures do not yet reach the bone but occasionally expand in cystic fashion into the deeper layers. The cartilage, subdivided into larger or smaller villi, resembles a sheepskin.

Grade 3: Now the fissures reach the bone which is exposed in areas of varying magnitude. In these areas a thickening or doubling of the calcification zone can be observed. Besides sclerosing of the subchondral bone, lacunar defects appear through which vascular connective tissue from the subcortical medullary spaces penetrates into the cartilage and decomposes it. Grade 3 of chondromalacia patellae thus represents a transitional step towards arthrosis.

A physically measurable loss of elasticity parallels the reduction in content of glycosaminoglycans (GAG) – and this not only in the tangential and transitional zones of the cartilage (which normally contain less GAG) but also in the perpendicular or pressure zone. During this process collagen fibrils, which are normally indistinguishable in the hyaline ground substance, become visible (unmasked) [13, 22, 28].

The chondrocytes act differently. Chondromalacia patellae grade 1 shows signs of increased activity (increase in cells, vacuolization); in grades 2 and 3, however, increasing degenerative changes are seen (edematous swelling, poorly stained nucleus, hypochromatosis).

Especially grade 3 is accompanied by secondary symptoms of chondrolysis. Frequently a chronic villous synovitis secondary to cartilage detritus exists [15]. In this case a tongue-shaped pannus can move from the synovial border forward to the center of the cartilage lesion. Small, shiny cartilage flakes can be detected in the usually somewhat increased, rather viscous but transparent synovial fluid (in aspiration of the joint this is diagnostically relevant).

The first chondromalacic foci are mostly situated in the proximal part of the medial articular facet or in the proximal part of the median ridge and, as a secondary step, spread to the lateral facet. Grinding grooves are frequently found directly opposite them on the femoral condyles as well as lamellar splittings of the articular cartilage.

Chondromalacia patellae must be distinguished from traumatic shearings of large flaps of cartilage, as Ganz and Wagner have described.

Accident Induced Damage of the Hyaline Articular Cartilage

Various accident-induced injurious agents can directly or indirectly affect the functional structure of the hyaline articular cartilage *at two points:*

1. By damaging the collagen fibrils in the tangential zone
2. By traumatically damaging the chondrocytes

In either case the compromise of the interconnecting system causes a loss in elasticity of the cartilage. The resulting nutritional disorder adds to the initial mechanical damage of the tissue. A secondary change in cellular secretion presumably causes the loss of GAG in the perpendicular zone. This in turn results in an additional reduction in elasticity of the intercellular substance itself.

This means that a trauma-induced damage of the fibrillar system or of the chondrocytes causes a vicious circle of pathogenetic factors, which eventually leads to progressive wear of the cartilage (Fig. 3) even under normal physiological strain.

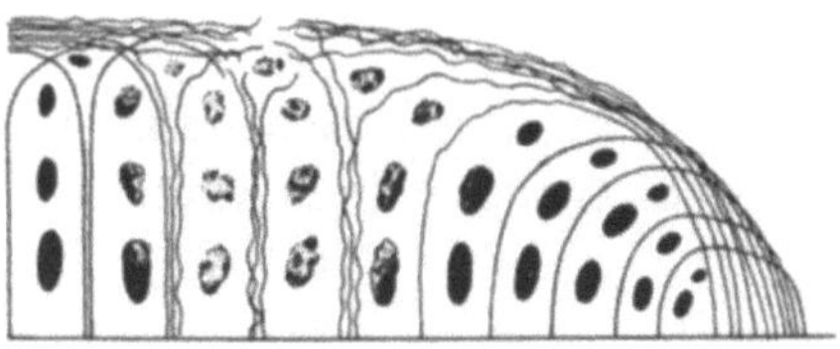

Fig. 3. Status after rupture of collagen fibrils in tangential zone and/or mechanical damage of chondroctytes. Fibrils slacken through rupture as well as loss of tension in chondrones. Mechanical wear caused by increased friction and nutritional deficiency caused by lack of elasticity accelerate degeneration

Thus we believe that the following injury mechanisms can produce cartilage damage which leads to cartilage wear as an initial stage.

1. Rupture of the Collagen Fibrils in the Tangential Zone

a) Vertical or violent pressure forces
b) Posttraumatic incongruence in the articular surface and correspondingly circumscribed areas with increased unit loads (pressure per cm^2)
c) Damage to the tangential fibre zone through proteolytic enzymes [17, 19]
d) Functionally increased unit load
e) Repetitive sub-threshold active loading (fatiguing) (23)

2. Damage to the Chondrocytes

a) Permanent pressure in a circumscribed area [2, 9, 17]
b) Impeded diffusion caused by a change in the synovial fluid
c) Mechanical cellular damage (either directly or through derangement of the surrounding intercellular substance)

Evaluation of the Isolated Injuries Which in Practice Directly or Indirectly Affect the Patellar Cartilage

In the following paragraphs we shall evaluate those injuries which are widely recognized as having etiologic importance that occur in practice and which, justly or unjustly, are held to be the cause of chondromalacia patellae.

Direct Contusion

A vertical blow on the patella caused by a fall or a sports accident can, depending on its direction and force, result in an initial rupture of the tangential fibres. A suddenly interrupted flexion of the knee joint in breaking a fall can lead not only to a traction fracture of the patella but also – as a late complication – to chondromalacia patellae.

The same applies to shearing forces that can be produced by a traumatic dislocation of the patella as a result of a torsion of the knee joint while it is stressed in flexion [18].

Examples: A 32-year old fireman suffered a lateral dislocation of the left patella at a moment when, standing in rubble, he slipped with his left foot while swinging a pickaxe. Intense pain set in together with a temporary effusion into the joint. After an initial improvement increasing localized pains appeared 2 years later inside the knee joint. Six years after the accident an arthrotomy showed a lesion of the meniscus, a chondromalacia patellae grade 3 and a shearing fracture on the lateral border of the lateral femoral condyle. Furthermore, there was chondromalacia of the articular cartilage in the trochlea.

On August 15 1973, a 35-year-old woman suffered a contusion of the left knee through a dashboard injury, together with other multiple contusions. After an initial improvement pains reappeared in the knee joint 6 weeks later and a plaster cast was applied for 2 months. After the cast was removed retropatellar pains persisted, especially while walking downhill. An arthrotomy was then carried out which revealed a chondromalacia grade 2 on the medial facet of the patella.

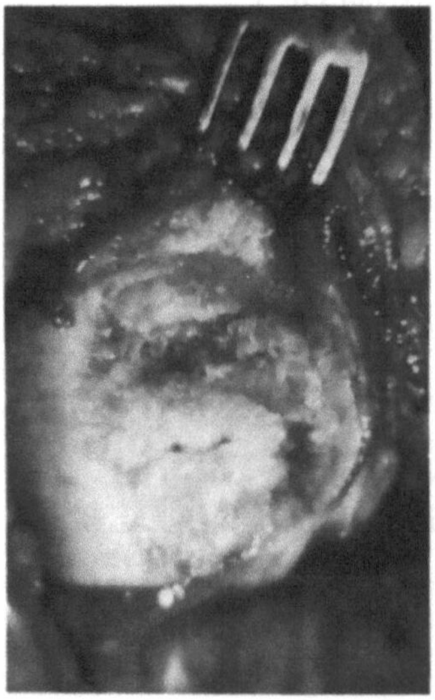

Fig. 4. Intraoperative condition of patella of L. W.: Chondomalacia grade 2 and 3, especially in the distal half of the patella; cartilage split in vertical fascicles and villi, also partly lifted off in discs

A 52-year-old patient, L. W., a nurse,[1] who had never had any complaints with her knee joints, suffered a violent collision of the right knee against an oxygen-transport apparatus in June 1973. Severe pains set in immediately and she was unable to work. X-ray showed no indication of a fracture. There was smooth swelling of the soft tissues

[1] I am indebted for this case to Dr. med. F. Schmid, chief of the surgical department, Bezirksspital Frutigen, who also operated on the patient.

but no effusion into the joint. Antiinflammatory agents freed the patient of her complaints within 10 days. Three months later the pains in the knee joint reappeared making a continued sitting position with flexed joint impossible. The pains especially increased in intensity when going up and down stairs. The patient spontaneously described a distinct grinding noise under the kneecap. The operation, which was carried out on 11-20-73 under the diagnosis of posttraumatic chondromalacia patellae, showed a typical chondromalacia grade 3, especially in the distal portion of the patella. The bone was partly exposed and the cartilage was partly split up into fascicles and threadlike formations. The most marked changes were found in the distal half of the patella and decreased proximally (Fig. 4). The trochlea of the femur showed a normal cartilage covering.

Chondromalacia patellae begins most commonly in the proximal half of the medial articular facet whence it gradually spreads laterally and distally. In this case the predominance of changes in the distal portion of the patella with a lessening toward the proximal portion speaks in favour of a traumatic etiology with damages to that portion of the patella which, independent of the demands of normal joint movement, had been affected by the injury. The integrity of the cartilage of the femoral joint suggested a short duration of the pathogenesis, as did the comparatively minimal synovitis described in the operative report.

Posttraumatic incongruence and functionally, produced zones of increased unit load: Intraarticular fractures, whose healing process causes step formation, produce circumscribed zones of higher unit load. It can hardly be disputed that these indirect consequences of accidents can cause a chondromalacia. Much harder to explain, however, are the chondromalacic damages occurring after fractures which are not in proximity to the joint (the femur or tibia shaft) as a consequence of healing in axial or rotatory union with corresponding abnormal tracking of the patella. The same applies to posttraumatic neuromuscular abnormalities.

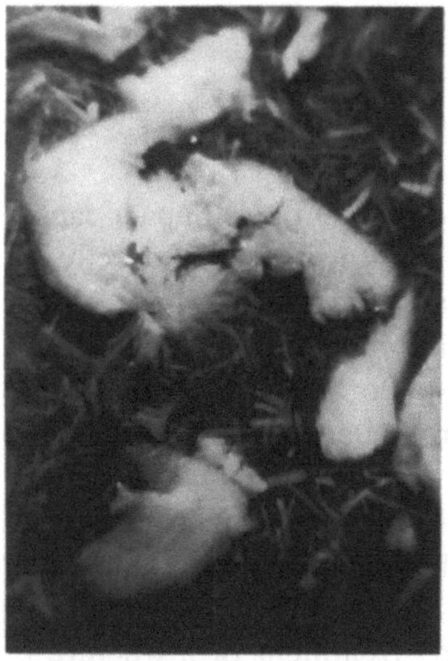

Fig. 5. Removed cartilage suspended in a physiological solution of saline. Severed parts of cartilage, delicate fragments as well as villous and lamellar sections, can be distinguished

Example: A 50-year-old man sustained a fracture of the femoral shaft in the proximal third. It was treated by internal fixation and healed in the correct position. As a consequence of iatrogenic damage to the innervation of the vastus lateralis chondromalacia patellae developed a year after the operation, resulting from a medial deviation of the kneecap from the trochlea.

Proteolytic damage to the tangential fibres through traumatic hemarthrosis. Chondromalacia patella which appears with a latent period of several months subsequent to a traumatic hemarthrosis that has been verified by aspiration, should, in our opinion, be recognized as accident-induced even if the particular kind of trauma does not suggest direct damage of the patellar cartilage.

The enzymatic damage of the cartilage through bloody effusions, as Cotta et al. have demonstrated, justifies further the requirement that posttraumatic hemarthrosis be treated with a prompt and complete evacuation of the joint through aspiration and irrigation, and, in recurring cases, through arthrotomy [7, 19].

Repetitive Sub-Threshold Loading

Clinical experience confirms the pathogenetic importance of such injurious agents, as for instance the frequent occurrence of chondromalacia patellae in soccer players and athletes in different sports [19, 24, 26]. The individual events, however, do not fall under the legal definition of an accident. However, since they lead to latent chondromalacia patellae and since this in turn can be transformed by a distinct injury into a clinically manifest state of pain, they deserve to be mentioned here. For purposes of expert medical opinion, they are not to be considered as the results of an accident but rather as a preexisting state in the sense of a knee condition peculiar to athletes [1].

Traumatic Damages of the Chondrocytes

An injury which, depending on the intensity and direction of its impact causes the tangential fibres to tear, will also damage the chondrocytes, be it directly, by mechanical destruction of their structure and derangement of the intercellular substance, or indirectly, through the above-mentioned nutritional disorder. Mechanically damaged chondrocytes will not be able to fulfill their task of maintaining the tension of the fibrils in the chondrone because of the reduction of intercellular pressure.

Trophic damage to the chondrocytes resulting from permanent compression of the cartilage in a circumscribed area is not easily recognizable as the indirect consequence of an accident. It occurs relatively frequently though with long periods of immobilization of the knee joint during treatment of a fracture or after injuries of the capsular ligament apparatus, especially when combined with a hemarthrosis. The same applies to posttraumatic paralyses or to posttraumatic Sudeck's atrophy (Fig. 6).

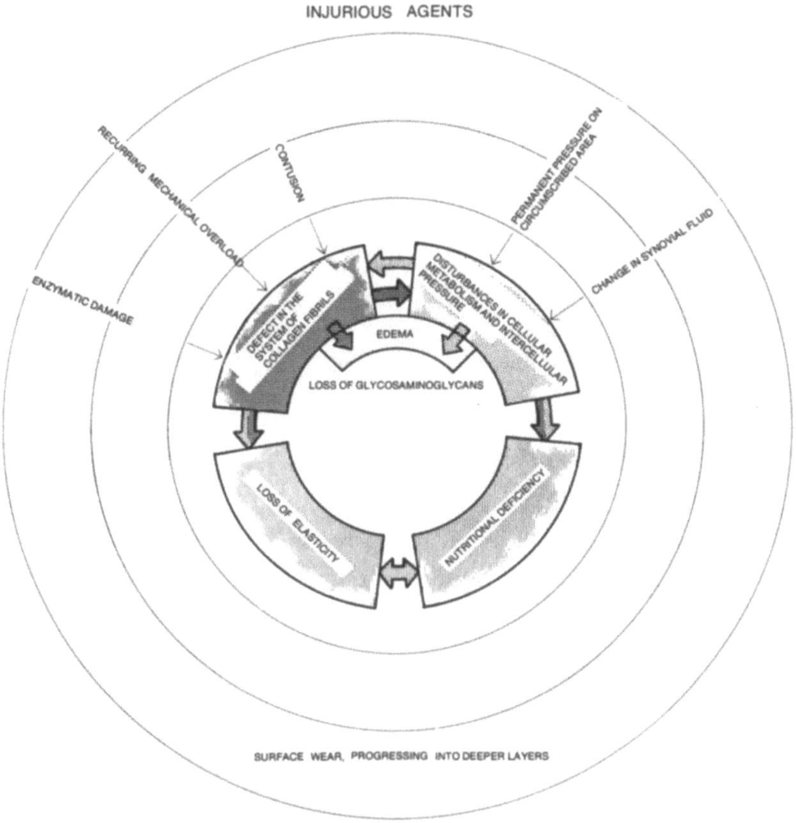

Fig. 6. Injurious agents – their manner and focus of attack with schematic representation of the interacting damaging influence of impaired structure and function

This presentation of the etiologic importance of isolated injury for the genesis of chondromalacia patellae is theoretical and needs further experimental confirmation. As a guideline it may facilitate the pathogenetic explanation and even the evaluation of specific cases. The recognition or rejection of chondromalacia patellae as resulting from an accident, based only on its clinical aspects, encounters two obstacles:

1. It must be stressed that chondromalacia patellae, resulting exclusively from an accident, manifests itself only after a certain latent period, namely when a *healthy* cartilage has suffered an injury which is what the definition of an "accident" requires. After the direct pain from the accident caused by contusion of skin and periosteum subsides, the wear of the cartilage requires a certain period of time until the clinical symptoms appear, especially since the pain of chondromalacia is mainly caused by secondary synovitis rather than by the injured cartilage itself.

2. The examiner must always take into consideration the entire complexity of the pathogenesis of chondromalacia patellae, which is compiled in Table 1. The forms resulting directly or indirectly from an isolated injury are framed in black. The table shows clearly that those resulting from trauma constitute only

Table 1. Pathogenesis of chondromalacia patellae and femoro-patellar arthrosis

Mechanical overload			*Disturbed regeneration*
Exogenous (trauma)		*Endogenous*	
Direct	*Indirect*		
Acute: Cartilage: Contusion Rupture (shearing) Bone: Fracture Patella, Condyles } Step-off Shaft, Condyles, Tibial-plateau } Axial or rotatory malposition	*Acute:* Sprain Hemarthrosis Posttraumatic immobilization and loss of movement	Dysplasia of patella Wiberg III Patella parva, magna partita *Malposition of patella* Chronic subluxation Recurrent dislocation Patella alta	1. *Change of synovia* Infection, hematogenic Posttraumatic Autotoxic Autoimmune reaction: RA
Chronic: Overload Sports Occupation Weight	*Chronic:* Posttraumatic neuro-muscular failings Posttraumatic Sudeck's disease	*Dysplasia of femoral condyles* Medial ridge Faulty rotation	2. *Changes in circulation* Arteriosclerosis Thrombosis Reflex sympathetic dystrophy (Sudeck's) 3. *Endocrine* Postmenopausal osteoporosis Hypothyroidism

about 50% of cases vs. endogenous-mechanical or tissue-trophic forms. Moreover it is possible that exogenous and endogenous excessive mechanical stress overlap or that autotoxic damages cause a predisposition of the cartilage for sub-threshold injury.

A causal evaluation of the injurious agents in question is difficult and requires a detailed knowledge of the etiology and pathogenesis of chondromalacia patellae as well as a thorough clinical and radiological examination of the entire damaged extremity.

Summary

Based on the functional structure of the hyaline articular cartilage, the direct or indirect precipitation of chondromalacia patellae through an accidental injury is illustrated. The possibility of asymptomatic, previously existing chondromalacic damage is pointed out as well as the latent period before clinical manifestations of a purely trauma-induced chondromalacia patellae. Pathogenetically contributing endogenous-mechanical or trophic factors are mentioned.

References

1. Aleman, O.: Acta chir. scand. **66,** 149 (1928)
2. Antoni, T.: J. Bone Jt Surg. **43 B,** 376 (1961)
3. Axhausen, G.: Virchows Arch. Path. Anat. **255,** 144 (1925)
4. Benninghoff, A.: Z. Zellforsch. **2,** H. 5 (1925)
5. Bethge, F. J. J.: Dtsch. med. Wschr. **87,** 636 (1962)
6. Büdinger, K.: Dtsch. Z. Chir. **92,** 510 (1908)
7. Cotta, H., Puhl, W.: H. Unfallheilk. **110,** 140 (1972)
8. Ekholm, R., Norbäck, B.: Acta orthop. scand. **21,** 82 (1951)
9. Ficat, P.: Pathologie fémoro-patellaire, Paris: Masson 1970
10. Fründ, H.: Zbl. Chir. **53,** 707 (1926)
11. Ganz, R.: H. Unfallheilk. **110,** 146 (1972)
12. Grueter, H.: Z. Orthop. **91,** 486 (1959)
13. Hirsch, C.: Acta chir. scand. Suppl. **83,** 1 (1944)
14. Landellis, J. W.: J. Bone Jt Surg. **39 B,** 584 (1957)
15. Hulten, O., Gellerstedt, N.: Acta chir. scand. **84,** 1 (1941)
16. Läwen, A.: Bruns' Beitr. klin. Chir. **134,** (1925)
17. Mathias, H. H., Glupe, J.: Arch. orthop. Unfall-Chir. **60,** 380 (1966)
18. Morscher, E.: Reconstr. Surg. Traumat. **12,** 2–26 (1971)
19. Noesberger, B.: Therap. Umschau **29,** 7, 424 (1972)
20. Outerbridge, R. E.: J. Bone Jt Surg. **43 B,** 752 (1961)
21. Owre, A.: Acta chir. scand. **77,** Suppl. 41 (1936)
22. Paul, B.: Med. Sport. **XIII,** 1, 13 (1973)
23. Radin, E. L., Paul, I. L.: Arthr. and Rheum. **14,** 356 (1971)
24. Schneider, G.: Arch. orthop. Unfall-Chir. **54,** 401 (1968)
25. Uehlinger, E.: H. Unfallheilk. **110,** 111 (1972)
26. Viernstein, R., Weigert, N.: Z. Orthop. **104,** 432 (1969)
27. Wagner, H.: H. Unfallheilk. **110,** 140 (1972)
28. Willes, Ph., Andrews, P. S., Dewas, H. B.: J. Bone Jt Surg. **42 B,** 95 (1960)

English translation from the German edition *Der Orthopäde,* Vol. 3, pp. 201–207 (1974),

Traumatic Injuries to the Articular Cartilage of the Knee

H. Wagner*

Traumatic injury to the articular cartilage of a joint commonly leads to degenerative arthrosis, thereby attaining clinical significance. Apart from the extent of the injury, the rate of development of the arthrosis is influenced by further factors. Cartilage injuries generally cannot be demonstrated radiologically, so that they are frequently recognized late if at all, and appropriate treatment is not instituted in time. Since articular cartilage has hardly any tendency to heal, the repercussions of isolated cartilage damage are further exacerbated. Those cartilage cells capable of division are situated in the tangential surface layer and are generally damaged by the injury. Even if they are preserved, they have only a limited capacity for proliferation. By formation of rounded complexes of cartilaginous tissues (cloning), they can only slightly reduce the defect from its margins. Even the regenerated tissue does not assume the ordered structure of the intact articular surface, so that the repair is always defective.

The poor healing ability of the hyaline cartilage tissue is also manifested in contusion injuries of the articular surface. Through the action of the high mechanical pressure, ruptures occur in the collagen fibrils, especially in the tangential layer. Mechanical damage to the chondrocytes also takes place. This combination of injuries brings about not only a loss in elasticity but also a disturbance in the nutrition of the articular cartilage in the affected area. The regenerative capacity of the unaffected chondrocytes is not sufficient to heal such a traumatic structural disruption of the joint cartilage. On the contrary, the contused area is further softened to some extent as a result of the nutritional disturbance brought about by the structural damage. The articular surface defect and the softened fibrillated areas of cartilage, which have resulted from the original injury, now serve to increase friction under load until finally radiologic evidence of arthrosis appears.

A healing of the defect by scar tissue formation is only to be expected if, in addition to the hyaline cartilage, the subchondral bone is included in the injury and the marrow space of the cancellous bone is opened. A functionally satisfac-

* Orthopädische Klinik des Wichernhauses (Head Physician: Prof. Dr. H. Wagner), Nuremberg/Altdorf, Federal Republic of Germany

tory fibro-cartilaginous scar can form from the invading granulation tissue. However, this hardly ever attains the quality of the natural joint surface.

The bleeding into the synovial space frequently observed in conjunction with the cartilage lesion, the post-traumatic effusion, and the reactive synovial pannus formation are further factors which increase the repercussions of the injury and can lead to a global enzymatic injury of the knee joint.

Finally, numerous mechanical factors also play a role in the chondral injury of the knee joint. Large defects in the main weight-bearing areas can bring about a rapid deterioration of the joint simply by reduction of available joint surface and by creating areas of high pressure point contact at the edges of the defect. Isolated fragments of the joint surface, as loose bodies in the joint, lead to recurring "locking" episodes which damage previously normal cartilage all the while sustaining the post-traumatic state of irritation of the joint. Painful locking episodes occur when flaplike cartilage fragments are lifted up at the edge of the defect. With repeated occurrences, smaller or larger fragments are broken off from these cartilage flaps. At arthrotomy, these are found distributed throughout the whole synovial space. Locking, painful movement, recurrent effusion, and limping caused by pain, finally lead to atrophy of both bone and the musculature frequently with an element of dystrophy included. All of these contribute to further acceleration of the post-traumatic arthrosis. Treatment by immobilization at this point can further enhance the negative effect of the disuse atrophy [5].

On the one hand one cannot count on the ability of the damaged cartilage to repair itself. On the other hand, the continuation of motion in the face of an intra-articular derangement, the disturbance of cartilage nutrition by hemarthrosis or post-traumatic effusion, the persistence of immobilization or inactivity leading to atrophy, all only serve to aggravate the injured state [3, 10, 11]. Our treatment must therefore be instituted early with a view to eliminating any obstacles to movement, whatever the nature of the original injury, and to normalizing the nutritional condition of the cartilage. A cicatrization of the articular surface defect, favorable to function, must be facilitated or the defects must be plugged by reimplantation of osteochondral fragments or, if necessary, also by transplantation. Restoration of joint function which is normal or near the normal creates the best conditions for overcoming a traumatic cartilage injury and for the prevention of post-traumatic arthrosis.

Traumatic damage to the cartilage of the knee joint may be the result of various mechanisms of injury. The possibilities for treatment and the prognosis depend on the kind and extent of the injury. In almost all injury mechanisms, there can be cartilage damage which is more or less restricted to the surface, or deeper cartilage-bone injuries.

1. Perforating Injuries of the Knee

The cartilage injury of the knee which is most easily understood in terms of mechanism and extent of injury is that resulting from perforating wounds caused by stabbing, a blow from an axe or other sharp-edged object. During the care which the wound itself necessitates, the cartilage lesion should already be identified. This should present no difficulties if the joint is inspected in the same degree of flexion in which it was injured. In smooth cut shearing injuries to the articular cartilage, no derangement of movement is anticipated. The detached cartilage fragments must simply be removed so that they do not cause any mechanical obstruction. Punched-out defects with sharp or frayed edges can lead to increased friction and post-traumatic inflammation, as well as to pinching of synovial folds. Defects with sharp edges must therefore always be smoothed.

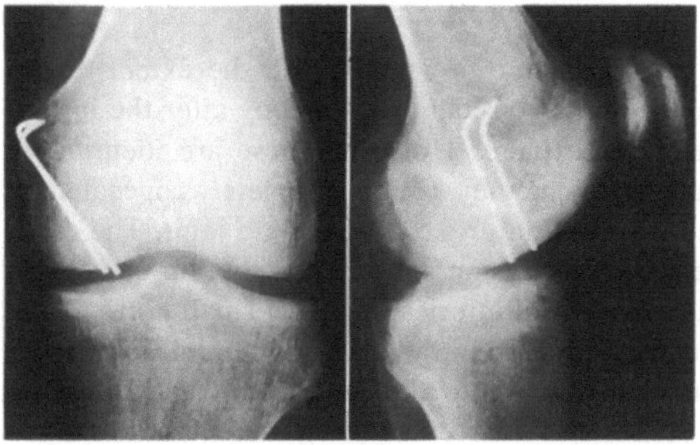

Fig. 1. Fixation of osteochondral fragments, osteochondrotic dissecates or osteocartilaginous transplants on the femoral condyle with Kirschner wires

Large detached osteochondral fragments should be replaced again in the defect as long as the conditions of the open joint wound allow. Fixation of the fragments with several Kirschner wires has proved satisfactory. The wires are drilled into the repositioned fragment from the articular surface to exit the bone again in the area of the epicondyles. The cut-off ends of the wire are countersunk just under the cartilage surface of the fragment. The opposite ends of the wire are bent back at the epicondyle and laid on the bone surface so that their position does not change (Fig. 1). After the fragments have healed, the wires can easily be removed again. There is no point in reimplanting large isolated parings of cartilage without a proportion of bone because these fragments do not heal. When a homologous or autologous cartilage transplantation appears appropriate in a large joint defect which cannot be restored, it should only be undertaken in a second sitting after the perforating wound has healed.

2. Contusion of Articular Cartilage

Contusion of articular cartilage occurs when corresponding articular bodies are pressed against one another with great force. In this mechanism of injury the cartilage tissue is crushed and its structure disrupted; collagen fibers and chondrocytes are torn, especially in the tangential layer. Under the action of excessive force, the surface of the articular cartilage ruptures. Stellate fissures, gaping tears, and crushing defects occur. The trauma when the kneecap strikes the dashboard, often in combination with a fracture of the neck of the femur or a fracture/dislocation of the hip joint, and a blow or fall on the kneecap with a bent knee joint, are typical examples of this mechanism of injury.

Contusion of the articular cartilage of the femoral condyle can also occur as a concomitant injury in tibial plateau fractures or from the lateral action of force on the extended knee which results in ligament rupture.

Symptoms

The clinical picture depends on the degree of severity and the extent of the cartilage injury and consequently varies considerably. Directly after the injury, the cartilage contusion causes intense pains. However, these are identifiable only in the isolated contusion injury since they can be completely concealed by the symptoms of a severe accompanying injury, e.g. of the hip joint. The cartilage contusion evokes an intense joint effusion and intense pain on movement already in the first hours. With superficial injuries involving small areas of the joint, the effusion and complaints subside in a few days and normal joint function eventually returns. Permanent damage to the joint is not anticipated in these cases, and the cartilage contusion is either not recognized at all or only at an arthrotomy carried out later and for another reason. If the contusion is more pronounced, the initial discomfort and effusion subside, only to reappear after a symptom-free period of 6 to 12 weeks after the injury. The patients often spontaneously report feeling friction when the joint is moved. Here arthrotomy reveals the typical cartilage lesion in the area of contusion. The surface has the dry, dull, fissured appearance of softened, yellow-colored cartilage, often with villous fronds floating above the surrounding surface. The synovial fluid contains many tiny fragments of cartilage. The synovial membrane appears hyperemic, edematous and proliferative. A synovial pannus which grows forward from the edge of the joint surface toward the center of the contused area is regularly encountered.

In severe contusion injuries in which tears and surface defects of the articular cartilage have already occurred during the initial injury, the symptom-free interval, characteristic of the milder forms of injury, does not take place. The initial intense pain and the synovial effusion also improve here, but pain on movement of the joint remains. The latter frequently leads to assumption of a meniscus lesion by the physician. Already after a short time, a capsule thickening develops with local hyperthermia. In testing movement of the knee joint, there is generally crepitus from the beginning. This crepitus increases markedly after 6–12 weeks. Now the X-ray (which is at first negative in all cartilage contusions) shows a demineralization of the bone which is maximal in the area of contusion, often with larger areas showing blurring of trabecular detail.

At arthrotomy, the local findings generally exceed those which the clinical and radiological picture would lead us to expect. In the area of contusion, there are deep tears, often with flaplike elevation of softened cartilage, and defects in the articular surface extending to the subchondral bone. The degree of the synovial inflammations with the pannus formation in the direction of the site of damage [15] is also striking. Evidently under the influence of the altered conditions within the joint, the articular cartilage which was not affected by the injury also shows a marked softening, even though the surface remains smooth. This can be appreciated by palpation of the articular cartilage with a blunt instrument. Such secondary changes are usually most pronounced on the posterior surface of the patella. This almost constant finding suggests that the cartilage of the patellar articular surface is especially sensitive to nutritional disturbances.

Therapy

Although pain and effusion are present, fresh cartilage contusion does not cause such prominent disturbances in joint movement that the degree of severity of the cartilage damage can be recognized from the clinical picture. Hence we do not consider an immediate arthrotomy to be advisable. With slight damage, the cartilage contusion cannot be diagnosed with certainty and in severe contusion its extent cannot be definitely assessed.

When the injury is fresh, bed rest must be maintained because of the pain. The leg should be elevated and supported by a foam splint. The articular effusion should be aspirated. Light compressive bandages and anti-inflammatory medication can favorably affect the soft tissue swelling and subsequent effusion. After subsidence of the acute pain, supervised range-of-movement exercises and isometric muscle exercises may be commenced; these should not exceed the pain threshold. The leg may assume a position of comfort in the foam splint which can lead to a fixed flexion contracture. This should be counteracted by placing the knee for several hours at a time in the fully extended position. Immobilization in a plaster cast should be avoided under all circumstances, because it only leads to further damage [5]. With increasing clinical improvement, the exercise program can be increased progressively. Weight-bearing exercises should only be begun cautiously with partial loading, checking for soft tissue swelling and pain.

In severe contusion injuries with persistent pain, swelling, and crepitus, arthrotomy is indicated after the third week. Shaving the frayed contusion area, the articular surface can be smoothed. This improves not only the tolerance to movement but also prevents the maintenance of synovial irritation on a mechanical basis. In areas of old contusion, the synovial pannus must also be removed. In extensive severe contusive injuries which extend to the bone, after shaving a softened cartilage layer, the subchondral bone can be perforated several times with a 2 mm drill. Cicatrization is then accelerated by the invasion of granulation tissue from the marrow space of the cancellous bone. Gentle but persistent movement in physiotherapy after the operation facilates a smooth fibrocartilaginous resurfacing which is favorable for function. On the other hand, if the leg is immobilized, irregular, flaplike sheets of scar tissue can form. The latter constitute a new hindrance to movement. If such deep foci of softening are situated in a major weight-bearing area of the articular surface, the involved site can also be replaced by a cartilage-bone transplant. In either case, normal weight bearing of the knee joint can be permitted only after 8 weeks at the earliest.

The surgical treatment of contusion injury to the articular surface of the knee joint which has been described may appear excessive to those less familiar with the subject. However, it must be realized that a large focus of softening of the articular surface always leads to arthrosis in a few years, while the surgical treatment can preserve the functional capacity of the knee joint for years.

3. Impression Fracture of the Articular Surface

Circumscribed fractures of the articular surface arise by the same mechanism of injury as the cartilage contusion injuries, i.e. violent compression of the corresponding joint surfaces on one another. In the impression fracture, the enveloping articular cartilage practically always remains intact. Therefore the question arises as to whether the individual differences in the strength of cartilaginous and bony tissues play a role, determining whether a cartilage contusion arises more readily in one case, and an impression fracture in another.

We distinguish three forms of osteochondral impression:

a) *The two-dimensional impression* is characterized by a circumscribed area of articular surface on the femoral condyle or on the tibial plateau which has sunk below the level of the joint surface. At the edge of the fragment, the otherwise intact articular surface shows a step-off, whose magnitude is directly proportional to the degree of the infraction.

Symptoms: The impression fracture is only slightly painful or not painful at all because the fragment is firmly rammed into the cancellous bone beneath it and is thus rigidly anchored. Crushing of the meniscus or a synovial fold occurring at the same time can themselves cause discomfort and further distract from the osteochondral injury. If there is no injury to soft parts, effusion and discomfort subside rapidly. Small joint step-offs escape clinical (and mostly also radiological) demonstration, while larger joint step-offs affect movement and occasionally cause pinching. The latter also show up on the X-ray pictures.

Treatment: Adequate treatment of small articular surface impressions consists of aspirating the synovial effusion and functional movement treatment with partial loading until the discomfort subsides. However, specific treatment is seldom instituted because as a rule the articular surface impression is first discovered when an arthrotomy is carried out because of accompanying injuries. When large step-offs are created in the articular surface, the osteochondral impression must be dealt with surgically because it otherwise leads to arthrosis. By raising the impression in the articular surface to the level of the surrounding cartilage and supporting it with a cancellous bone graft, the effect of the injury can be eliminated.

b) The *springy osteochondral impression* has only been observed by us in osteoporotic femoral condyles. Under the action of force, the articular surface is dented in, causing a compression fracture of cancellous bone. The intact articular surface then returns to its initial form, so that a flat hollow space remains behind under the subchondral plate. These fractures are very painful because the affected articular surface is always indented again on any attempt to move the knee.

Symptoms: In the forefront of the clinical picture is the intense pain and sensitivity of the affected condylar section to pressure. Pain can also be elicited by digital pressure on the condyle in the flexed knee. An articular effusion and capsular swelling can regularly be demonstrated on the affected side. Since the radiological finding is negative, this relatively rare lesion is generally only verified by arthrotomy.

Treatment: In theory, the pain on movement and the springy compressibility of the articular surface can be eliminated by a supporting cancellous bone graft. However, one is reluctant to undertake such an intervention in most older patients, especially since a reliable stabilization of the articular surface is certainly not simple technically with the general atrophy of the cancellous bone even in the deeper layers of the femoral condyle. For this reason, we have always preferred conservative treatment, and, after aspiration of the synovial effusion, have always carried out supervised range of movement exercises and partial loading up to the pain threshold. After 4–6 weeks, the complaints improve, although months can pass before there is complete resolution of the discomfort.

c) The *articular edge impression on the femoral condyle* was already mentioned by Budinger in 1906 (2) and very comprehensively described a few years ago by Morscher [7–9]. The injury arises as a result of forced hyperextension of the knee joint: in the hyperextended position the anterior edge of the tibial

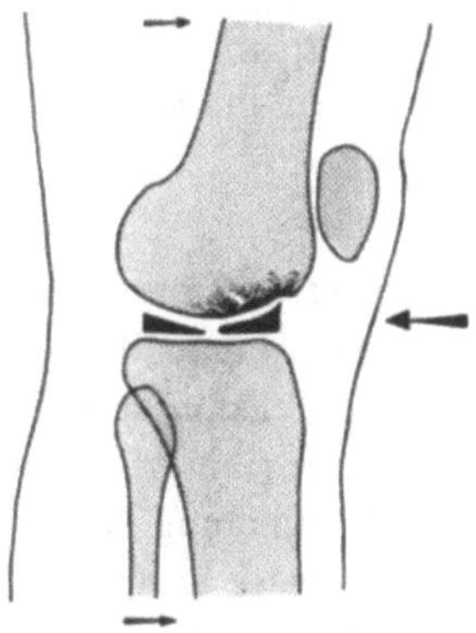

Fig. 2. Articular edge impression in the femoral condyle in hyperextension injury of the knee joint [8]

plateau or the base of the meniscus is pressed into the femoral condyle where it leaves behind a relatively sharp-edged groove with intact articular cartilage (Figs. 2 and 3). At the same time, a crushing of the meniscus also often occurs at this point, leading to fibrous thickening. When the knee joint is extended, the scarred thickened edge of the meniscus catches in the dent in the femoral condyle and is squeezed between the femoral condyle and the anterior edge of the tibial head. This elicits pain and leads to chronic inflammation of the joint. The impression in the femoral condyle and the base of the anterior horn of the meniscus form, so to speak, the two arms of a forceps in which fatty tufts of the infrapatellar fat pad can be pinched on extension of the knee. Through this mechanism of repetitive internal trauma, a state of synovial irritation is maintained with a fingerlike pannus formation running along the impression in the femoral condyle. In the 13 cases of this type of injury in which we have opened the joint, cicatrization of the anterior horn of the meniscus, an abnormality of the fat pad and synovial pannus formation were encountered routinely. Such findings were demonstrable ten times on the medial and three times on the lateral femoral condyle. In one case, an impression of the medial femoral condyle also additionally resulted in a rupture of the anterior transverse ligament.

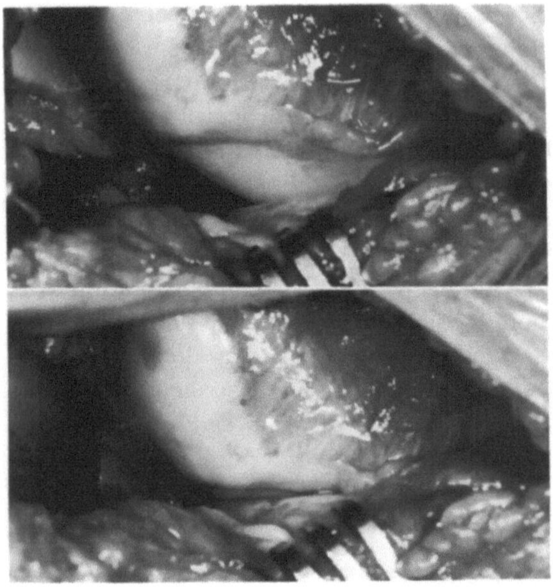

Fig. 3. Articular edge impression on the medial femoral condyle, on the right, after hyperextension injury of the knee in a 35-year-old man. In the upper half of the picture (slight bending of the knee joint), the sharp angular articular surface impression with synovial pannus formation is recognizable. In the lower half of the picture (almost complete bending of the knee joint), the anterior edge of the tibial head dips into the dent in the femoral condyle

Symptoms: A description of the mechanism of injury is instructive for recognition of the type of injury which has occurred. Most patients unequivocally describe a hyperextension injury. Subsequently, intense pain on extension and effusion characterize the clinical state. After subsidence of the acute pain, the terminal few degrees of extension remain painful. Episodes of "pinching something" in the joint during extension are frequently mentioned. These temporarily increase the pain on extension. There may frequently be pain on palpation of the anterior joint line on the affected side in the area of the meniscus and the tibial plateau, but not the femoral condyle. The infrapatellar fat pad may also be tender to touch, but not in the femoral condyle. The radiological examination contributes little information: Localized osteoporoses to the margins of the joint are frequently present, while the impression fracture itself is only rarely unequivocally recognizable.

Therapy: The painful limitation of extension in this type of injury is so clear that it justifies an immediate arthrotomy to eliminate the derangement of movement. It is of primary importance to smooth the relatively sharp-edged depression in the femoral condyle so that the meniscus and fat body can no longer be pinched here, but slide over the area. Since the anterior edge of the impression groove is not included in the normal range of movement of the tibial femoral joint, there is no objection to excision of this cartilage ledge to the level of the impression, thereby producing a smooth transition to the anterior condylar section. Any traumatized fibrosed pad should also be excised and the thickened anterior meniscus horn should be reduced to normal height by tangential excision. We do not consider that resection of the otherwise intact meniscus is advisable. Finally, in the case of an old injury, the synovial pannus must also be removed.

4. Tangential Shearing off of Articular Cartilage

Patella dislocation is the classic injury in which shearing at the knee gives rise to a traumatic cartilage injury. Especially in the position of flexion of the knee joint in which dislocation usually occurs, the lateral stability of the patella is ensured extraordinarily well by the groovelike configuration of the trochlea of the femur and by the tension on the joint capsule and the quadriceps muscle. The action of a very violent force is necessary to dislocate the patella laterally out of this groove. In patellar dislocation, these substantial forces accordingly result in shearing stress applied to the articular surface of the patella and trochlea. These forces are strongest in the moment in which the median edge of the patella jerks over the sharp-angled edge of the lateral femoral condyle. As this happens, cartilage or osteochondral fragments from the median edge of the patella and the angle of the lateral femoral condyle can be broken off. At the same time, a rupture of the medial retinacular capsule also occurs, which enhances the potential for recurrent dislocation. The injury leads to an acute hemarthrosis with intense pain on movement of the joint as well as swelling and stretching pain of the articular capsule. The sheared-off fragments of the patella and the femoral condyle can cause blocking of the knee, but primarily a block to extension.

Tangential shell-like shearing off of cartilage at the femoral condyle occurs much more rarely in rotation or torsional trauma of the bent knee [4]. In such an injury which came under our care, the 16-year-old patient described the mechanism of injury very characteristically. He had stepped in a frozen tire track, the foot rotated medially inward, stuck in the track while he twisted laterally, falling on the bent knee. There was a loud cracking sound in the knee joint and he immediately had very severe pain. In the subsequent aspiration, 80 cm^3 of pure blood were obtained.

Symptoms: All fresh cartilage disruptions have in common the intense pain and massive articular hemorrhage. Most also demonstrate immediately a derangement of movement with catching or restriction of extension. In patellar dislocation, the median edge of the patella is especially sensitive to pressure. Sometimes, a defect can be palpated in the disrupted medial retinaculum. When the articular cartilage of the femoral condyle has been sheared off, the maximum tenderness is localized to the joint line. The X-ray shows the osseous portions of the fragments, which are generally located in the suprapatellar pouch, in the intercondylar notch or above the anterior edge of the tibial plateau. Purely cartilaginous fragments are, of course, not visible in the X-ray.

In the case of old cartilage shearing injuries, there is, as a rule, capsular swelling and the frequent finding of dystrophy of the soft parts in the knee-joint region. The thigh musculature is atrophic and the knee is held slightly flexed. Movement is restricted in both directions with pain at the extremes of movement. The X-ray now shows marked, diffuse osteoporosis with poor definition of the joint margins in some parts. The sheared-off cartilage fragments are now often distinctly recognizable because the cartilage tissue has taken up calcium salts.

Therapy: Tangential cartilage shearing injuries should always immediately be treated surgically. At the very least, the blood should be removed from the synovial space by aspiration. A satisfactory result of treatment cannot be achieved without arthrotomy because the raw defects in the articular surfaces and the fragments lying free in the synovial space lead to persistent derangement of motion and to further severe damage of the knee joint. At the arthrotomy, the defects in the articular surfaces are smoothed and the free fragments removed. In patellar dislocation, it will hardly ever be necessary to reimplant fragments. However, suturing of the ruptured medial retinaculum is required to avoid recurrent dislocation.

In the shell-like shearings from the femoral condyle, the fragments are probably always purely articular cartilage. These must be removed so that they do not cause any interference with motion. There is no point in reimplantation because the fragments have no osseous basis and therefore will not heal. The articular surface defects located in the main weight-bearing zone on the femoral condyle should be repaired with an osteochondral transplant [14]. The articular surface is less capable of resistance to wear if left to spontaneous fibrocartilaginous cicatrization.

5. Chronic Cartilage Damage in Persistent or Recurrent Locking Episodes

In the course of time, persistent derangement of joint movement, especially recurrent locking episodes from a damaged meniscus or loose bodies, lead to extensive uni- or multifocal areas of cartilage damage and formation of defects in the cartilaginous articular surface. The chronic, recurrent synovitis with effusion existing at the same time leads to nutritional disturbances and diminution in the elasticity of the hyaline articular cartilage. In turn, this exacerbates the mechanical damage to the articular surface. Finally, the reactive synovial pannus results in the disruption of the structural organization of the articular cartilage and leads to degenerative joint disease. Cartilage damage of this sort is especially pronounced in high-performance athletes who persist unrelentingly in their training after a meniscus injury (Fig. 4). Here meniscus fragments are rubbed, frayed and rounded off between the articular surfaces, so that in spite of the severe joint damage a remarkably good function remains for a long time, as long as the cartilage reserve is sufficient, i.e. as long as the articular surfaces are still covered by a cartilage covering. However, as soon as the bony articular bodies rub directly against each other, increasing joint complaints appear. Especially severe mechanical cartilage injuries can also occur if the knee is forcefully manipulated in the presence of a locked knee due to a meniscus tear or if it is immobilized in a plaster cast because of persistence of the locking.

Symptoms: After the "catching" and locking episodes have persisted for years with chronic recurring effusions, the cartilage damage shows clinically and radiologically the picture of degenerative arthrosis with capsular thickening and pain on movement and loading of the joint. The medial half of the joint is often more affected, so that a secondary varus deformity has also developed through the loss of medial articular cartilage.

Therapy: In the damaged knee joint, treatment can often save very little and basically it must deal with the arthrosis. In demonstrable locking episodes, blocks to movement can be removed, but often an osteotomy to correct an axial deformity, which has already set in, is the treatment of choice. This picture of chronic cartilage attrition is perhaps the best argument for the importance of surgically eliminating intra-articular blocks to movement at an early stage.

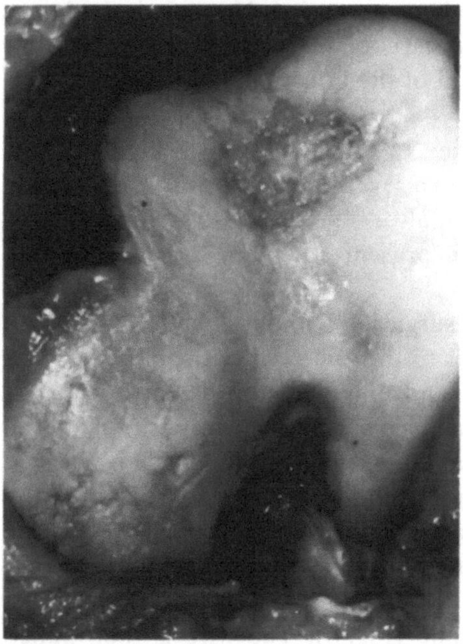

Fig. 4. Chronic cartilage wear in the left knee joint of a 32-year-old athlete, 10 years after lesion of the medial meniscus with recurrent locking episodes

6. Traumatic Osteochondrosis Dissecans

Several authors have described the traumatic genesis of an osteochondrosis dissecans [1, 6–9, 12, 13]. Morscher [7–9] has pointed out that the traumatic genesis must be considered above all for osteochondrosis dissecans of the lateral femoral condyle. In our patient material, we have not yet seen among our own patients a traumatically induced osteochondrosis dissecans. However, we have seen several cases of osteochondrosis dissecans in which a malformed lateral meniscus would fold forcefully up into the osteochondritic defect as the knee was extended. This also speaks for the mechanical induction on the defect.

Symptoms and Therapy: According to the literature, the syndrome of traumatic osteochondrosis dissecans (with the exception of the localization) resembles the condition which has arisen non-traumatically. Once the fragment has separated, any loose bodies must be removed and the edges of the defect smoothed. In osteochondrotic defects in portions of the articular surface on which there is great weight bearing, reimplantation of the dissecates or plugging of the defect with an osteochondral transplant is advisable.

7. Cartilage Avulsion Injury

A special form of articular cartilage injury is observed in ligamentous tears in childhood. Because of the incomplete degree of ossification of the cartilaginous anlage of the joint, not only the ligament insertion (as in the adult) but also large parts of the adjacent articular surface are also torn. Typical of this injury is the cruciate ligament tear in childhood due to hyperextension. Not only is the intercondylar eminence avulsed but also large parts of the articular surface of the tibial plateau are torn. However, the extent of the injury cannot be appreciated radiologically (Fig. 5).

Symptoms: The avulsion injury involving the tibial plateau leads to a firm block to extension of the knee in addition to a severe hemarthrosis. The anterior drawer sign which is always present cannot always be demonstrated because of the severe pain and tense effusion often present when the patient presents acutely.

Therapy: The injury should be treated surgically without delay, as this is the only way of preventing permanent injuries to the knee. After opening the joint from the median parapatellar approach and emptying the hemarthrosis, the avulsed fragment of the intercondylar eminence can easily be repositioned. The fragment can be fixed very reliably with a thin Kirschner wire which is inserted three to four fingerbreadths below the joint line on either the medial or the lateral surface of the tibia and drilled in a cranial direction through the repositioned intercondylar eminence. The cranial end of the wire is bent in the form of a hook with a small pliers. In certain cases, the attachment of the anterior cruciate ligament can be included at the same time (Fig. 6). The wire is then pulled

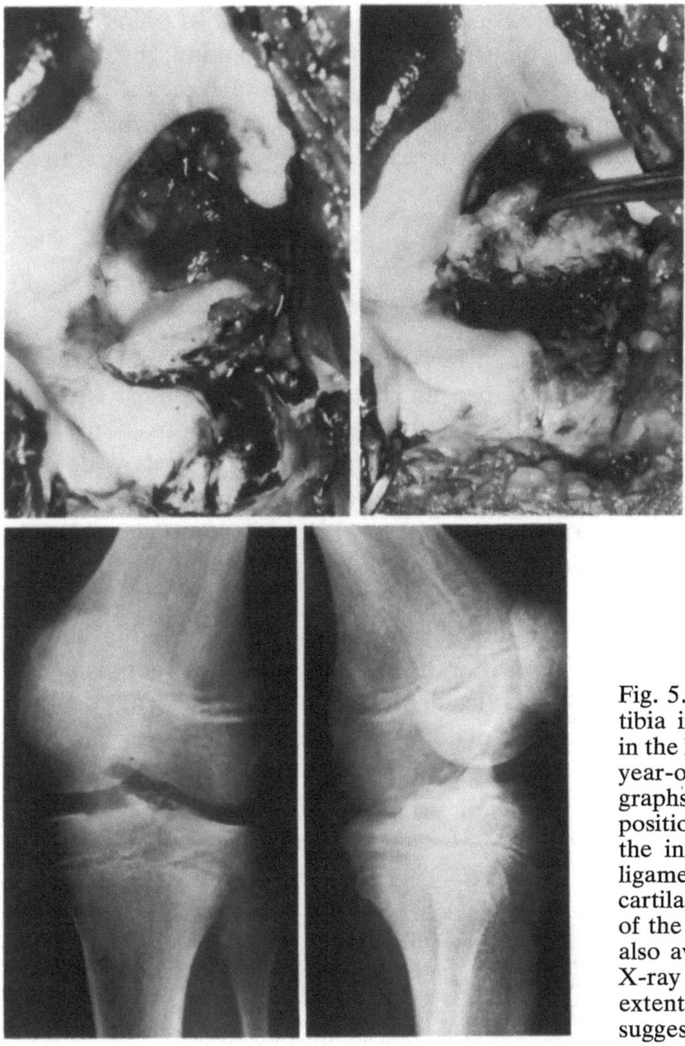

Fig. 5. Avulsion injury of the tibia intercondylar eminence in the left knee joint of an 11-year-old girl. The two photographs on the left show the position at operation: with the insertion of the cruciate ligament, a large part of the cartilaginous articular surface of the medial tibial plateau is also avulsed. On the oblique X-ray of the knee joint, the extent of the injury is only suggested

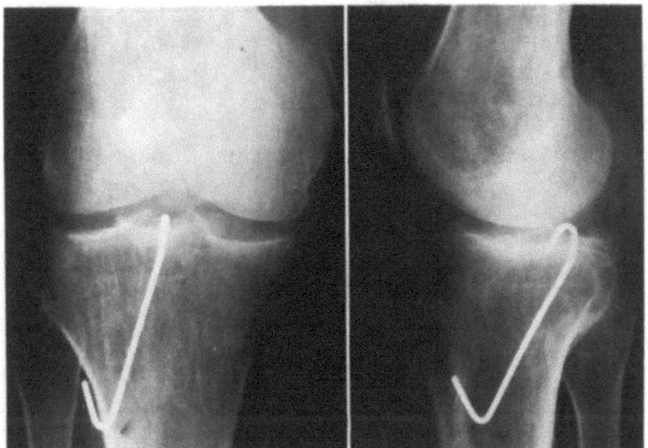

Fig. 6. Fixation of the torn intercondylar eminence with a Kirschner wire bent round into a hook.

strongly back through and bent back in a cranial direction at its point of entry into the tibia and cut off. Besides the simple and reliable fixation, the thin wire has the advantage that it does not damage the epiphyseal plate of the proximal tibia. This surgical repositioning is followed by active exercises in which above all a fixed flexion contracture is to be avoided. The Kirschner wire is removed again after 3 months.

Summary

Injuries to the cartilaginous articular surface lead to arthrosis. Its repercussions can be reduced only by timely diagnosis and treatment. Since most cartilage injuries escape radiological demonstration, they are often overlooked although they are based on a characteristic mechanism of injury and they show definite clinical symptoms, especially in the knee. Intense pain, effusion and bleeding into the joint as well as intra-articular derangement in movement and gliding in the absence of a radiological finding should always suggest the possibility of a traumatic cartilage injury.

The most important concern of therapy is to remove the effusion or hemarthrosis into the joint. In disturbances of movement, surgical treatment is necessary to smooth the uneveness in the articular surface, to replace fractured osteochondral fragments in position and, if need be, to plug large defects in the articular surface with transplants.

References

1. Aichroth, P. M.: J. Bone Surg. B **51,** 181 (1969)
2. Büdinger, K.: Dtsch. Z. Chir. **84,** 311 (1906); cited by Morscher and Pfeiffer [9]
3. Cotta, H., Puhl, W.: H. z. Unfallhk. **110,** 152 (1972)
4. Ganz, R.: H. z. Unfallhk. **110,** 146 (1972)
5. Matthiass, H. H., Glupe, J.: Arch. orthop. Unfallchir. **60,** 380 (1966)
6. May, E., Kuhn, D., Diethelm, L.: Arch. orthop. Unfallchir. **54,** 301 (1962)
7. Morscher, E.: Orthop. Praxis **6,** 31 (1970)
8. Morscher, E.: Reconstr. Surg. Traumat. **12,** 2 (1971)
9. Morscher, E., Pfeiffer, K. M.: Z. Unfallmed. u. Berufskrankh. **1,** 47 (1970)
10. Puhl, W., Dustmann, H. O., Schulitz, K.-P.: Z. Orthop. **109,** 475 (1971)
11. Puhl, W., Dustmann, H. O.: Z. Orthop. 110, **42** (1972)
12. Smillie, I. S.: J. Bone Surg. B **39,** 248 (1957)
13. Smillie, I. S.: Osteochondrosis Dissecans. Loose Bodies in Joints. Etiology, Pathology, Treatment. Edinburgh, London: E. & S. Livingstone 1960
14. Wagner, H.: Z. Orthop. **98,** 333 (1964)
15. Wagner, H.: H. z. Unfallhk. **110,** 140 (1972)

English translation from the German edition of *Der Orthopäde,* Vol. 3, pp. 208–216 (1974),

Subject Index

List of Contributors

Bandi, Prof. Dr. W.
Chirurgische Abteilung, Regionalspital, CH-3800 Interlaken, Switzerland

Eichler, Prof. Dr. J.
Mosbacher Straße 10, D-6200 Wiesbaden, Federal Republic of Germany

Figner, Dr. G.
Orthop. Universitäts-Klinik, Felix-Platter-Spital, Burgfeldstraße 101,
CH-4000 Basel, Switzerland

Heidensohn, Dr. P.
Orthopädische Klinik und Poliklinik der Universität, Rathsberger Straße 57,
D-8520 Erlangen, Federal Republic of Germany

Raymond E. Hogue, Ph. D.
School of Related Health Professions, University of Mississippi, School of
Medicine, 1350 E. Woodrow Wilson Drive, Jackson, Mississippi 39216, USA

Hohmann, Prof. Dr. D.
Orthop. Univ.-Klinik, Waldkrankenhaus, Rathsberger Strasse 57,
D-8520 Erlangen, Federal Republic of Germany

James L. Hughes, Jr. M. D.
Division of Orthopaedic Surgery, University of Mississippi, Medical School,
Jackson, Mississippi, USA

Kieser, Dr. Ch.
Chirurgische Klinik, Stadtspital Triemli, CH-8063 Zurich, Switzerland

Meyer, E.
Direktor der Bundesfachschule für Orthopädie-Schuhtechnik, Ricklinger
Stadtweg 92, D-3000 Hanover, Federal Republic of Germany

Morscher, Prof. Dr. E.
Orthopädische Universitäts-Klinik, Felix-Platter-Spital, Burgfeldstraße 101,
CH-4000 Basel, Switzerland

Müller, Dr. W.
Orthopädische Klinik, Kantonsspital, CH-4000 Basel, Switzerland

Petersen, Prof. Dr. D.
Orthopädische Klinik der Krankenanstalt Herzogin-Elisabeth-Heim,
Leipziger Str. 24, D-3300 Braunschweig-Melverode,
Federal Republic of Germany

Rüttimann, Prof. Dr. A.
Institut für Röntgendiagnostik, Chirurgische Klinik, Stadtspital Triemli,
CH-8063 Zürich, Switzerland

Wagner, Prof. Dr. H.
Orthopädische Klinik des Wichernhauses, Postfach 22, D-8503
Altdorf, Federal Republic of Germany

Weigert, Prof. Dr. M.
Krankenhaus Am Urban, Abt. f. Orthopädie und Traumatologie,
Dieffenbachstr. 1, D-1000 Berlin 61

MIX
Papier aus verantwortungsvollen Quellen
Paper from responsible sources
FSC® C105338

If you have any concerns about our products,
you can contact us on
ProductSafety@springernature.com

In case Publisher is established outside the EU,
the EU authorized representative is:
Springer Nature Customer Service Center GmbH
Europaplatz 3, 69115 Heidelberg, Germany

Printed by Libri Plureos GmbH
in Hamburg, Germany